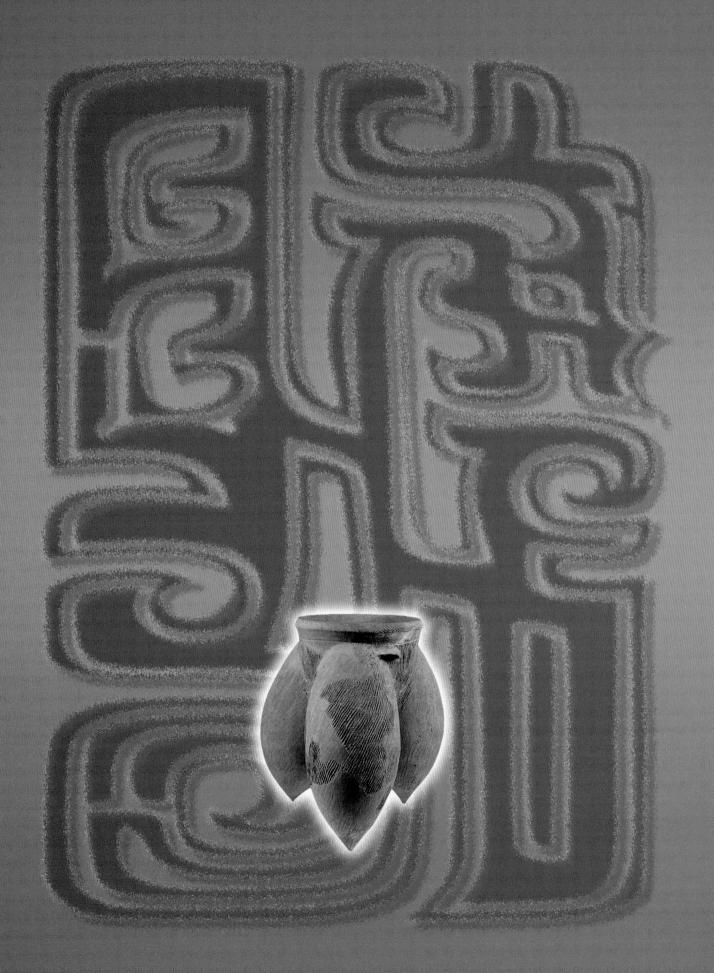

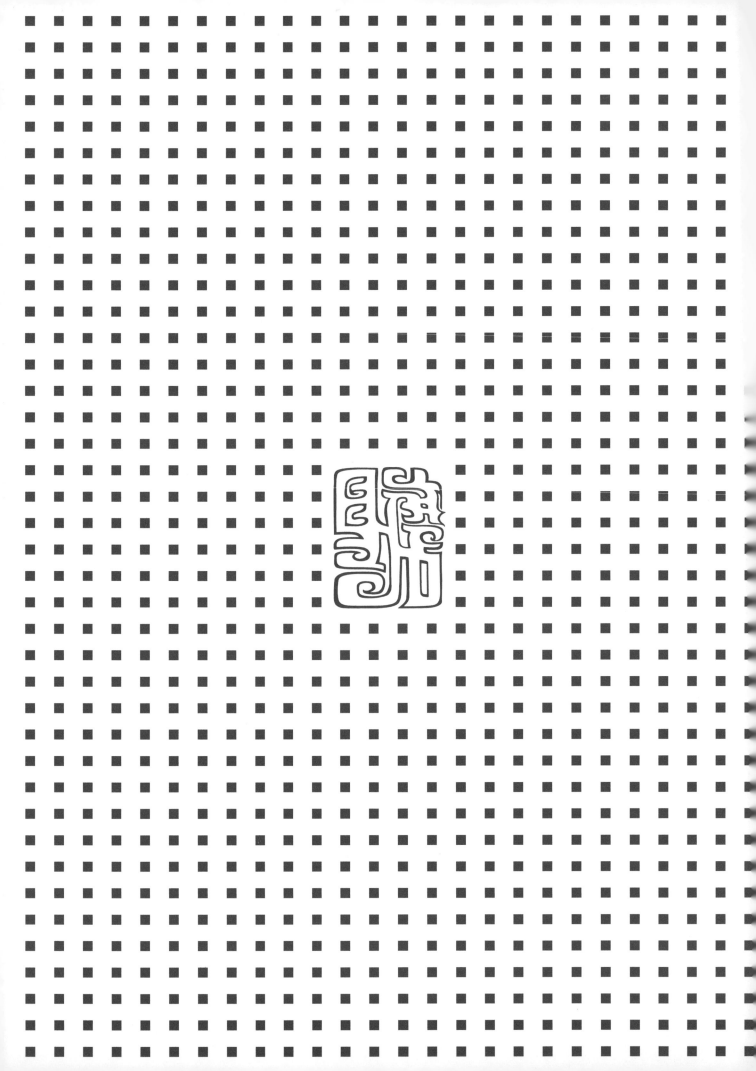

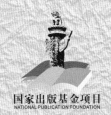

国家出版基金项目
NATIONAL PUBLICATION FOUNDATION

中华医药卫生

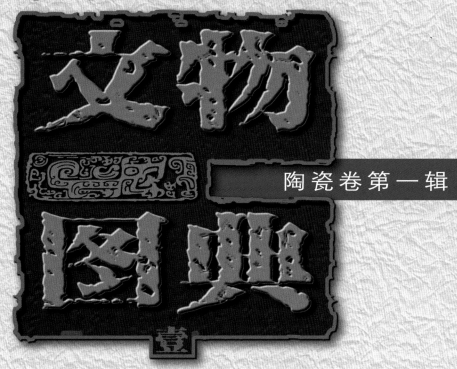

陶瓷卷第一辑

主　编　李经纬　梁　峻　刘学春
总主译　白永权
主　译　陈向京

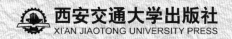

西安交通大学出版社
XI'AN JIAOTONG UNIVERSITY PRESS

图书在版编目 (CIP) 数据

中华医药卫生文物图典 .1. 陶瓷卷 . 第 1 辑 . / 李经纬，
梁峻，刘学春主编 .— 西安：西安交通大学出版社，2016.12
ISBN 978-7-5605-7028-0

Ⅰ . ①中… Ⅱ . ①李… ②梁… ③刘… Ⅲ . ①中国医药学—
古代陶瓷—中国—图集 Ⅳ . ① R-092 ② K870.2

中国版本图书馆 CIP 数据核字（2015）第 022424 号

书　　名　中华医药卫生文物图典（一）陶瓷卷第一辑

主　　编　李经纬　梁　峻　刘学春

责任编辑　李　晶

出版发行　西安交通大学出版社

　　　　　（西安市兴庆南路 10 号　邮政编码 710049）

网　　址　http://www.xjtupress.com

电　　话　（029）82668805 82668502（医学分社）

　　　　　（029）82668315（总编办）

传　　真　（029）82668280

印　　刷　中煤地西安地图制印有限公司

开　　本　889mm×1194mm　1/16　印张 21.25　字数 333 千字

版次印次　2017 年 12 月第 1 版　2017 年 12 月第 1 次印刷

书　　号　ISBN 978-7-5605-7028-0

定　　价　680.00 元

读者购书、书店添货、如发现印装质量问题，请通过以下方式联系、调换。

订购热线：（029）82665248　（029）82665249

投稿热线：（029）82668805　（029）82668502

读者信箱：medpress@126.com

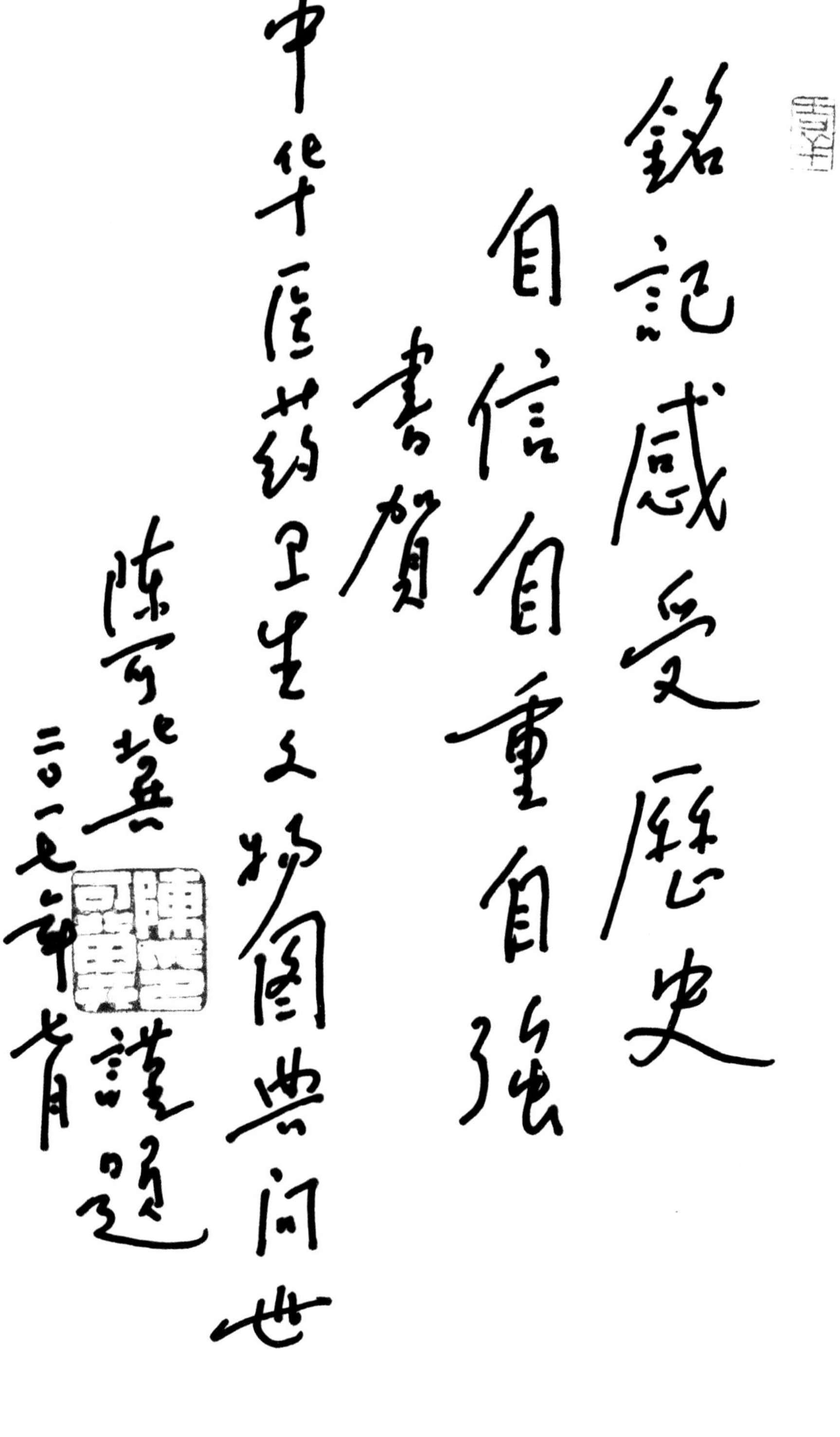

铭记感受历史

自信自重自强

书贺

中华医药卫生文物图典问世

陈可冀 谨题

二〇一六年肖月

陈可冀　中国科学院院士、国医大师

精修醫藥衛生文物

圖典功著當代

深究岐黃學術思想

淵源惠澤千秋

中華醫藥衛生文物圖典出版誌慶

丁酉孟秋 孫光榮 敬題於北京

孫光荣　国医大师

中華醫藥衛生文物圖典出版

彰顯中醫藥
文化精神

体現中醫藥
歷史价值

歲次丁酉夏　王琦

王琦　国医大师

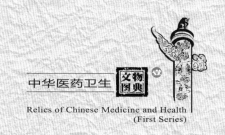

中华医药卫生文物图典（一）
丛书编撰委员会

主　编　李经纬　梁　峻　刘学春

副主编　廖　果　吴鸿洲　康兴军　和中浚　刘小斌　杨金生

　　　　　郑怀林　徐江雁　白建疆　黄　煌

编　委　李洪晓　梁永宣　王强虎　董树平　马　健　王　霞

　　　　　张雅宗　朱德明　包哈申　张建青　郑　蓉　庄乾竹

　　　　　李宏红　刘哲峰　王宏才　陈润东

总主译　白永权

主　译　陈向京　聂文信　范晓晖　温　睿　赵永生　杜彦龙

　　　　　吉　乐　李小棉　郭　梦　陈　曦

副主译（按姓氏音序排列）

　　　　　董艳云　姜雨孜　李建西　刘　慧　马　健　任宝磊

　　　　　任　萌　任　莹　王　颇　习通源　谢皖吉　徐素云

　　　　　许崇钰　许　梅　詹菊红　赵　菲　邹郝晶

译 者（按姓氏音序排列）

迟征宇　邓　甜　付一豪　高　琛　高　媛　郭　宁

韩　蕾　何宗昌　胡勇强　黄　鋆　蒋新蕾　康晓薇

李静波　刘雅恬　刘妍萌　鲁显生　马　月　牛笑语

唐云鹏　唐臻娜　田　多　铁红玲　佟健一　王　晨

王　丹　王　栋　王　丽　王　媛　王慧敏　王梦杰

王仙先　吴耀均　席　慧　肖国强　许子洋　闫红贤

杨姣姣　姚　晔　张　阳　张　鋆　张继飞　张梦原

张晓谦　赵　欣　赵亚力　郑　青　郑艳华　朱江嵩

朱瑛培

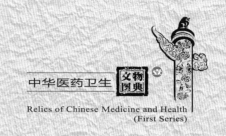

中华医药卫生文物图典

Relics of Chinese Medicine and Health
(First Series)

本册编撰委员会

主　编　李经纬　梁　峻　刘学春

副主编　廖　果　吴鸿洲　康兴军　和中浚　刘小斌　杨金生
　　　　　郑怀林　徐江雁　白建疆　黄　煌

编　委　李洪晓　梁永宣　王强虎　董树平　马　健　王　霞
　　　　　张雅宗　朱德明　包哈申　张建青　郑　蓉　庄乾竹
　　　　　李宏红　刘哲峰　王宏才　陈润东

总主译　白永权

主　译　陈向京

副主译　许　梅

译　者　邹郝晶　董艳云　刘妍萌　高　媛　王　晨
　　　　　郑艳华　王梦杰　张晓谦　王　丽　许子洋

丛书策划委员会

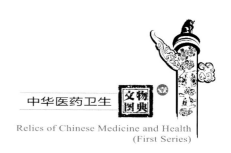

中华医药卫生
文物图典

Relics of Chinese Medicine and Health
(First Series)

序 言

　　探索天、地、人运动变化规律以及"气化物生"过程的相互关系，是人类永恒的课题。宇宙不可逆，地球不可逆，人生不可逆业已成为共识。天地造化形成自然，人类活动构成文化。文物既是文化的载体，又是物化的历史，还是文明的见证。

　　追求健康长寿是人类共同的夙愿。中华民族之所以繁衍昌盛，健康文化起了巨大的推动作用。由于古人谋求生存发展、应对环境变化产生的智慧，大多反映在以医药卫生为核心的健康文化之中，所以，习总书记说："中医药学是中国古代科学的瑰宝，也是打开中华文明宝库的钥匙"。

　　秉持文化大发展、大繁荣理念，中国中医科学院李经纬、梁峻等为负责人的科研团队在完成科技部"国家重点医药卫生文物收集调研和保护"课题获 2005 年度中华中医药学会科技二等奖基础上，又资鉴"夏商周断代工程""中华文明探源工程"等相关考古成果，用有重要价值的新出土文物置换原拍摄质量较差的文物，适当补充民族医药文物，共精选收载 5000 余件。经西安交通大学出版社申报，《中华医药卫生文物图典（一）》（以下简称《图典》）于 2013 年获得了国家出版基金的资助，并经专业翻译团队翻译，使《图典》得以面世。

　　文物承载的信息多元丰富，发掘解读其中蕴藏的智慧并非易事。　医药卫生文物更具有特殊性，除文物的一般属性外，还承载着传统医学发展史迹与促进健康的信息。运用历史唯物主义观察发掘文物信息，善于从生活文物中领悟卫生信息，才能准确解读其功能，也才能诠释其在民生健康中的历史作用，收到以古鉴今之效果。"历史是现实的根源"，任何一个民族都不能割断历史，史料都包含在文化中。"文化是民族的血脉，是人民的精神家园"，文化繁荣才能实现中华民族的伟大复兴。值本《图典》付梓之际，用"梳理文化之脉，必获健康之果"作为序言并和作者、读者共勉！

中央文史研究馆馆员
中国工程院院士　　王永炎

丁酉年仲夏

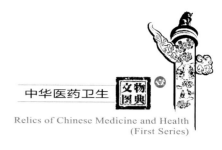

中华医药卫生 文物图典

Relics of Chinese Medicine and Health
(First Series)

前 言

　　文化是相对自然的概念，是考古界常用词汇。文物是文化的重要组成部分，既是文明的物证，又是物化的历史。狭义医药卫生文物是疾病防治模式语境下的解读，而广义医药卫生文物则是躯体、心态、环境适应三维健康模式下的诠释。中华民族是56个民族组成的多元一体大家庭，中华医药卫生文物当然包括各民族的健康文化遗存。

　　天地造化如造山、板块漂移、气候变迁、生物起源进化等形成自然。气化物生莫贵于人，即整个生物进化的最高成果是人类自身。广义而言，人类生存思维留下的痕迹即物质财富和精神财富总和构成文化，其一般的物化形式是视觉感知的文物、文献、胜迹等。其中质变标志明晰的文化如文字、文物、城市、礼仪等可称作文明。从唯物史观视角观察，狭义文化即精神财富，尤其体现人类精、气、神状态的事项，其本质也具有特殊物质属性，如量子也具有波粒二相性，这种粒子也是物质，无非运动方式特殊而已。现代所谓可重复验证的"科学"，事实上也是从文化中分离出来的事项，因此也是一种特殊文化形式。追求健康长寿是人类共同的夙愿。中华民族之所以繁衍昌盛，是因为健康文化异彩纷呈。中华优秀传统医药文化之所以博大精深，是因为其原创思维博大、格物致知精深，所以，习总书记说："中医药学是中国古代科学的瑰宝，也是打开中华文明宝库的钥匙"。

文化既反映时代、地域、民族分布、生产资料来源、技术水平等信息，又反映人类认知水平和生存智慧。发掘解读文物、文献中蕴藏的健康知识和灵动智慧，首先是从事健康工作者的责任和义务。《易经》设有"观"卦，人类作为观察者，不仅要积极收藏展陈文物，而且要善于捕捉文物倾诉的信息，汲取养分，启迪思维，收到古为今用之效果。墨子三表法，首先一表即"本之于古者圣王之事"，也是强调古代史实的重要性。"历史是现实的根源"，现实是未来的基础。任何一个国家、地区、民族都不能割断历史、忽略基础，这个基础就是文化。"文化是民族的血脉，是人民的精神家园"。文化繁荣才能驱动各项事业发展，才能实现中华民族的伟大复兴。

人类从类人猿分化出来。"禄丰古猿禄丰种"是云南禄丰发现的类人猿化石，距今七八百万年。距今 200 万年前人类进入旧石器时代，直立行走，打制石器产生工具意识，管理火种，是所谓"燧人氏"时代。中国留存有更新世早、中期的元谋、蓝田、北京人等遗址。距今 10 万—5 万年前，人类进入旧石器时代中期，即早期智人阶段，脑容量增加，和欧洲、非洲人种相比，原始蒙古人种颧骨前突等，是所谓"伏羲氏"时代。中国发现的马坝、长阳、丁村人等较典型。距今 5 万—1 万年前，人类进入旧石器时代晚期，即晚期智人阶段，细石器、骨角器等遍布全国，山顶洞、柳江、资阳人等较典型。

中石器时代距今约 1 万年，是旧石器时代向新石器时代的短暂过渡期，弓箭发明，狗被驯化。河南灵井、陕西沙苑遗址等作为代表。距今 1 万—公元前 2600 年前后，人类进入新石器时代，磨光石器、烧制陶器，出现农业村落并饲养家畜，是所谓"神农氏"时代。公元前 7000 年以来，在甲、骨、陶、石等载体上出现契刻符号、七音阶骨笛乐器等，反映出人文气息趋浓。公元前 6000—公元前 3500 年的老官台、裴李岗、河姆渡、马家浜、仰韶等文化遗址，彰显出先民围绕生存健康问题所做的各种努力。

公元前 4800 年以来，以关中、晋南、豫西为中心形成的仰韶文化，是中原史前文化的重要标志。以半坡、庙底沟类型为典型，自公元前 3500 年走向繁荣，属于锄耕粟黍稻兼营渔猎饲养猪鸡经济方式，彩陶尤其发达。公元前 4400—公元前 3300 年，长江中游的大溪文化，薄胎彩陶和白陶发达。公元前 4300—公元前 2500 年山东丰岛的大汶口文化，红陶为主。公元前 3500 年前后，辽东的红山文化原始宗教发展。公元前 3300 年以来，长江下游由河姆渡、马家浜文化衍续的良渚文化和陇西的马家窑文化、江淮间的薛家岗文化时趋发达。

公元前 2600—公元前 2000 年，黄河中下游龙山文化群形成，冶铸铜器，制作玉器，土坯、石灰、夯筑技术开始应用。公元前 2697 年，轩辕战败炎帝（有说其后裔）、蚩尤而为黄帝纪元元年。黄帝西巡访贤，"至岐见岐伯，引载而归，访于治道"。其引归地"溱洧襟带于前，梅泰环拱于后"，即今河南新密市古城寨。岐黄答问，构建《黄帝内经》健康知识体系，中华文明从关注民生健康起步。颛顼改革宗教，神职人员出现；帝喾修身节用，帝尧和合百国，舜同律度量衡，大禹疏导治水，中华民族不断繁衍昌盛。

公元前 2070 年，禹之子启以豫西晋南为中心建立夏王朝，二里头青铜文化为其特征，半地穴、窑洞、地面建筑并存。饮食卫生器具、酒器增多。朱砂安神作用在宫殿应用。公元前 1600 年，商灭夏。偃师商城设有铸铜作坊。公元前 1300 年，盘庚迁殷，使用甲骨文。武丁时期青铜浑铸、分铸并存。公元前 1056 年，相传周"文王被殷纣拘于姜里，演《周易》，成六十四卦"。公元前 1046 年，武王克商建周，定都镐京。青铜器始铸长篇铭文，周原发掘出微型甲骨文字。公元前 770 年，平王东迁。虢国铸铜柄铁剑。公元前 753 年，秦国设置史官。公元前 707 年出现蝗灾、公元前 613 年出现"哈雷彗星"，均被孔子载入《春秋》。公元前 221 年，秦始皇统一中国，多元一体民族大家庭形成，中华医药卫生文物异彩纷呈。

中国是治史大国，历来重视发展文化博物事业，1955 年成立卫生部中医研究院时就设置医史研究室，1982 年中国医史文献研究所成立时复建中国医史博物馆研究收藏展陈文物。2000—2003 年，经王永炎院士、姚乃礼院长等呼吁，科技部批准立项，由李经纬、梁峻为负责人的团队完成"国家重点医药卫生文物收集调研和保护"项目任务，受到科技部项目验收组专家的高度评价，获中华中医药学会科技进步二等奖。2013 年，在国家出版基金资助下，课题组对部分文物重新拍摄或必要置换、充实民族医药文物后，由西安交通大学出版社编辑、组聘国内一流翻译团队英译说明文字付梓，受到国家中医药博物馆筹备工作领导小组和办公室的高度重视。

"物以类聚"，《图典》主要依据文物质地、种类分为 9 卷，计有陶瓷，金属，纸质，竹木，玉石、织品及标本，壁画石刻及遗址，少数民族文物，其他，备考等卷。同卷下主要根据历史年代或小类分册设章。每卷下的历史时段不求统一。遵循上述规则将《图典》划分为 21 册，总计收载文物 5000 余件。对每件文物的描述，除质地、规格、馆藏等基本要素外，重点描述其在民生健康中的作用。对少数暂不明确的事项在括号中注明待考。对引自各博物馆的材料除在文物后列出馆藏外，还在书后再次统一列出馆名或参考书目，以充分尊重其馆藏权，也同时维护本典作者的引用权。

21 世纪，围绕人类健康的生命科学将飞速发展，但科学离不开文化，文化离不开文物。发掘文物承载的信息为现实服务，谨引用横渠先生四言之两语："为天地立心，为生民立命"，既作为编撰本《图典》之宗旨，也是我们践行国家"一带一路"倡议的具体努力。希冀通过本《图典》的出版发行，教育国人，提振中华民族精神；走向世界，为人类健康事业贡献力量。

李经纬　梁峻　刘学春

2017 年 6 月于北京

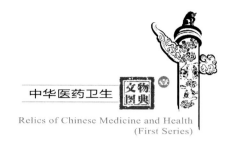

中华医药卫生 文物图典

Relics of Chinese Medicine and Health
(First Series)

目 录

第二章 夏商周

第三章　春秋战国

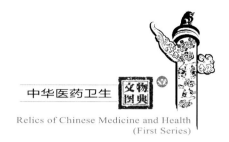

中华医药卫生
Relics of Chinese Medicine and Health
(First Series)

contents

Chapter Two　　Xia Shang Zhou

Chapter Three   Spring and Autumn Period and Warring States Period

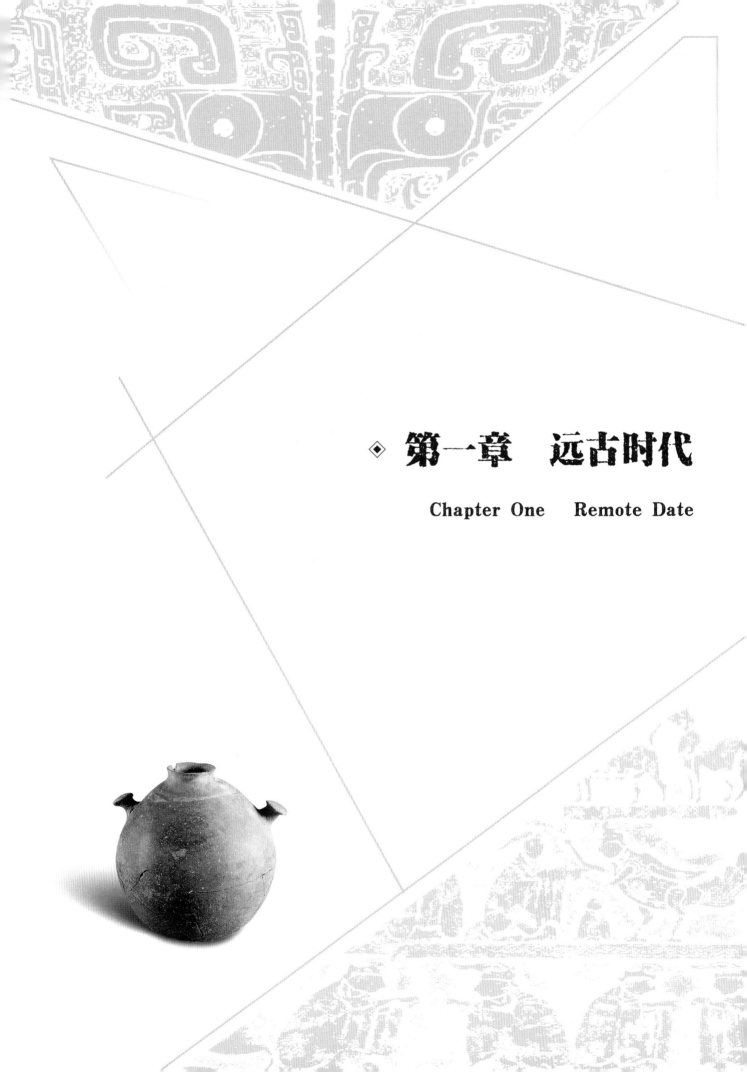

第一章 远古时代

Chapter One　Remote Date

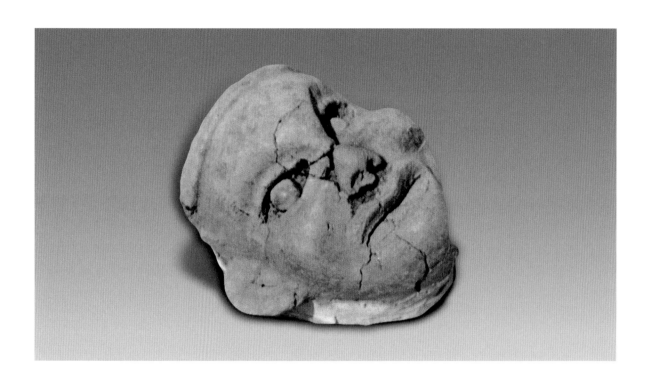

彩塑女神头像

新石器时代

泥塑

宽 16.5 厘米，高 22.5 厘米

Painted Head Sculpture of Goddess

Neolithic Age

Clay

Width 16.5 cm/ Height 22.5 cm

1983 年于辽宁省牛河梁红山文化遗址出土。此头像反映当时我国的巫职人员已经作为特定阶层出现。

辽宁省博物馆藏

It was excavated at the Niuheliang Archaeological Site of Hongshan Culture in Liaoning Province in the year 1983. The head sculpture suggests that practitioners of witchcraft have appeared as a special social class at that time in China.

Preserved in Liaoning Provincial Museum

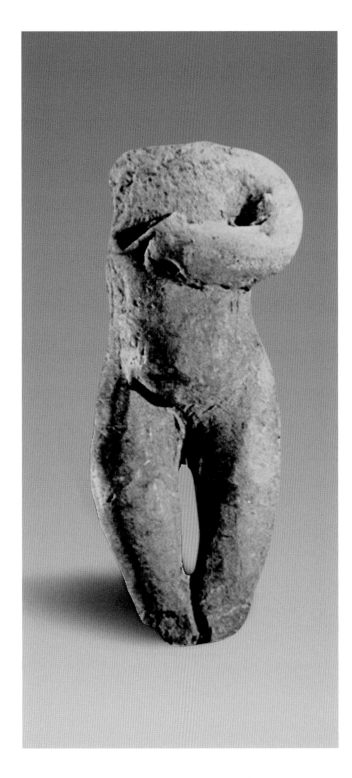

陶塑孕妇

新石器时代

陶质

残高 7.8 厘米

Pottery Figure of Pregnant Woman

Neolithic Age

Pottery

Residual Height 7.8 cm

该藏距今 5000 多年。1982 年辽宁喀左东山
嘴出土。体态修长，上身前倾，左手贴于上腹。
体型、性别特征明显。

中国国家博物馆藏

This object is believed to have a history of
approximately 5,000 years. It was excavated
from Dongshan Zui at Kazuo County, Liaoning
Province in the year 1982. The woman has a
slender figure, with the upper body leaning
forward and the left hand placed on the upper
part of the abdomen. This figure shows obvious
gender and physical characteristics.
Preserved in National Museum of China

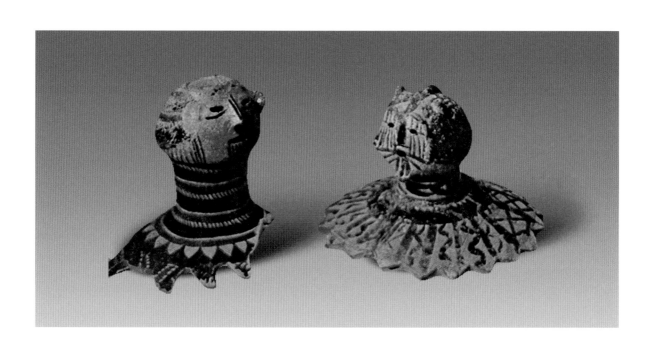

人头形陶器盖

新石器时代
陶质
左：高 15 厘米
右：高 13 厘米
该藏距今 4500 年左右。甘肃东乡出土。

瑞典东方博物馆藏

Pottery Lids in the Shape of Human Head

Neolithic Age
Pottery
Left: Height 15 cm
Right: Height 13 cm
These pottery lids were made some 4,500 years ago. It was excavated from Dongxiang County in Gansu Province.
Preserved in Museum of Far Eastern Antiquities

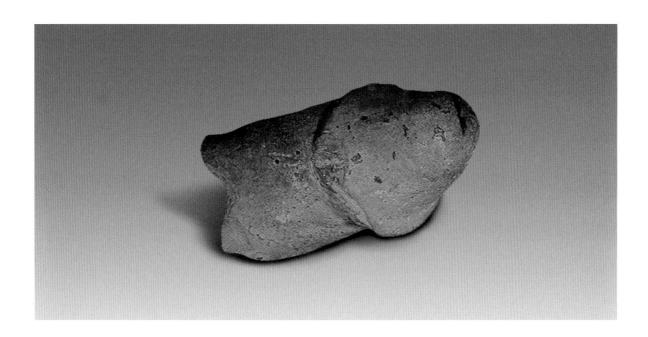

陶祖

新石器时代

陶质

残长 7.5 厘米

江苏省南京锁金村遗址北路北草地出土。

南京博物院藏

Pottery Male Genital

Neolithic Age

Pottery

Residual Length 7.5 cm

This object was unearthed from North lawn of North road at Suojin Village in Nanjing, Jiangsu Province.

Preserved in Nanjing Museum

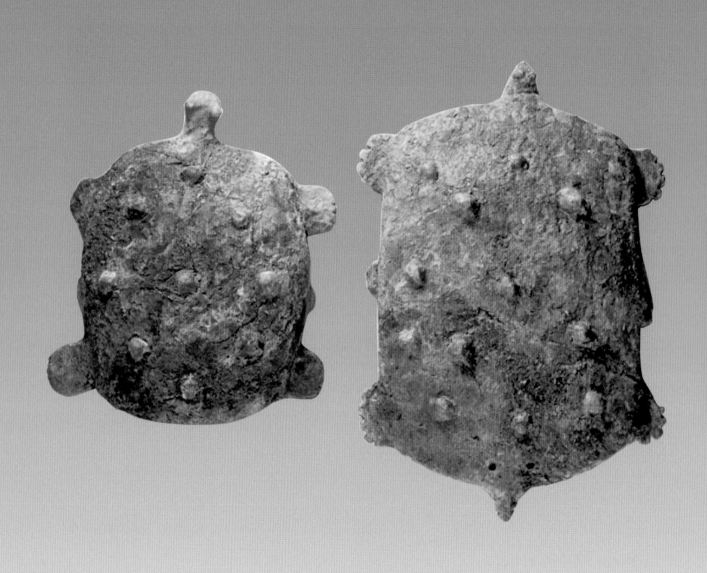

陶龟

崧泽文化

陶质

右龟：长 25.8 厘米，宽 17.4 厘米，高 3.6 厘米

均为泥质黑皮陶，一大一小。大的略呈方形，头尖有尾。小的呈椭圆形，头圆无尾。两龟都有六只脚,还在背甲上分别堆塑了十一枚(大)和九枚(小)乳钉状凸起。出土时两只龟腹部相合，放置于墓主的腿脚部位。

浙江省文物考古研究所藏

Pottery Tortoises

Songze Culture

Pottery

Right: Length 25.8 cm/ Width 17.4 cm/ Height 3.6 cm

The two tortoises, one being slightly bigger than the other, were made of black clay pottery. The bigger one is square in shape, with a pointed head and a tail; the smaller one is oval in shape, with a rounded head but no tail. Both of the tortoises have six feet. The dorsal surfaces of the carapace are covered with moulded designs of papillae, eleven on the big one and nine on the small one. The abdomens of the two tortoises were placed together when excavated, and they were put besides the legs of the master in the tomb.

Preserved in Institute of Cultural Relics and Archaeology of Zhejiang Province

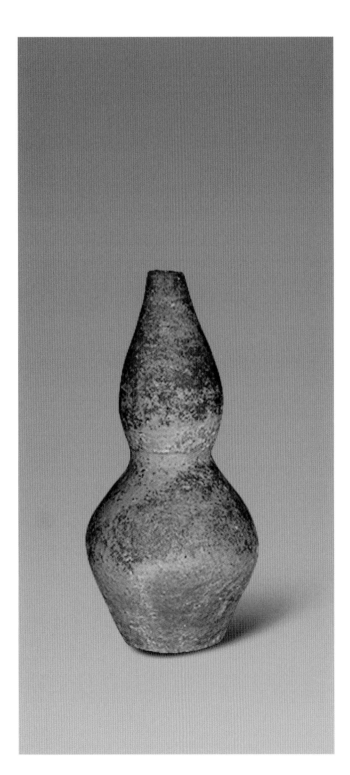

葫芦瓶

新石器时代

夹砂红陶质

口径 2 厘米，底径 6.8 厘米，通高 23 厘米，
重 700 克

Gourd-shaped Vase

Neolithic Age

Red Sandy Pottery

Mouth Diameter 2 cm/ Bottom Diameter 6.8 cm/

Height 23 cm/ Weight 700 g

小口葫芦状，平底，无纹饰，夹粗砂红陶。
盛贮器。完整无损。

陕西医史博物馆藏

The gourd-shaped vase features a small mouth
and a flat bottom without any decoration on the
body. It was made of red sandy pottery. The
vase was utilized as a container. It is kept intact.
Preserved in Shaanxi Museum of Medical History

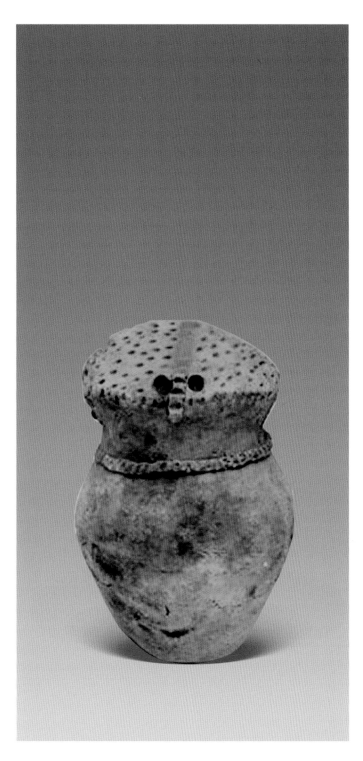

鸮面罐

新石器时代（齐家文化）

夹砂陶质

口径 10.5 厘米，底径 7 厘米，高 18.5 厘米

Jar with Design of Owl Head

Qijia Culture, Neolithic Age

Sandy Pottery

Mouth Diameter 10.5 cm/ Bottom Diameter

7 cm/ Height 18.5 cm

口部有两个滤孔，可用于煎煮药物。通体造型与今柳湾所用之煎药砂锅十分相似。青海柳湾出土。

青海柳湾彩陶博物馆藏

There are two filtration slit pores on the mouth of the jar. It can be used to decoct Chinese traditional medicine. The design of the jar is similar to the ceramic pots used for preparing herbal decoction in present Liuwan Village.It was excavated from Liuwan Village in Qinghai Province.

Preserved in Liuwan Painted Pottery Museum, Qinghai Province

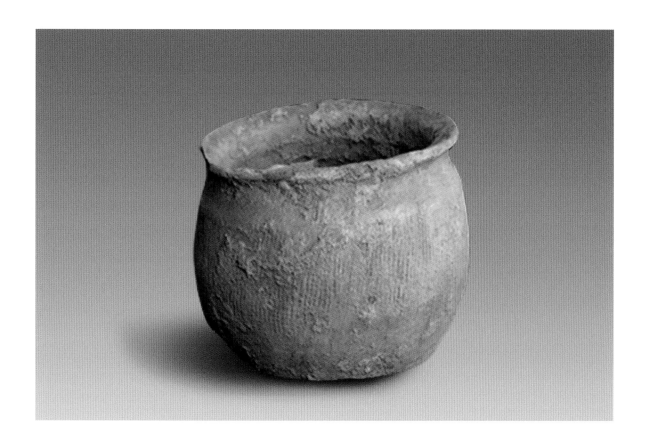

陶罐

龙山文化

陶质

口径 10 厘米，底径 7.6 厘米，高 8.6 厘米，重 350 克

Pottery Jar

Longshan Culture

Pottery

Mouth Diameter 10 cm/ Bottom Diameter 7.6 cm/ Height 8.6 cm/ Weight 350 g

敞口，直腹，平底，腹部饰细绳纹。盛贮器。

口沿残。陕西省澄城县征集。

陕西医史博物馆藏

This pottery jar, a storage container, has a flared mouth, a flat bottom and a straight abdomen decorated with thin cord patterns. The jar, with the mouth rim cracked, was collected from Chengcheng County, Shaanxi Province.

Preserved in Shaanxi Museum of Medical History

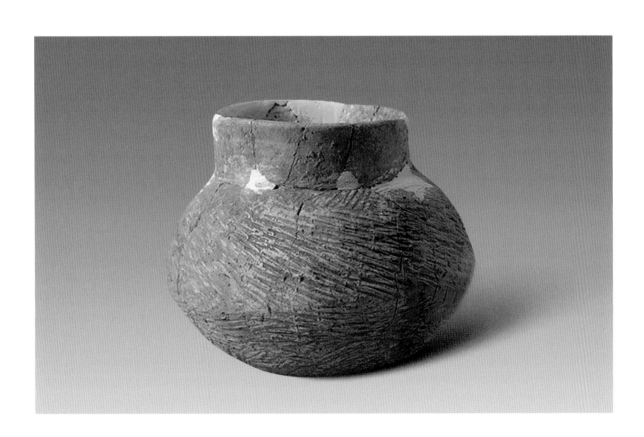

泥质灰陶罐

马桥文化

灰陶质

口径 8 厘米，高 10 厘米

Grey Clay Pottery Jar

Maqiao Culture

Grey Pottery

Mouth Diameter 8 cm/ Height 10 cm

1997 年浙江遂昌好川墓地出土。

遂昌县文物管理委员会藏

The jar was excavated from Haochuan Cemetery at Suichang County, Zhejiang Province.
Preserved in Department of Cultural Relics Coneservation of Suichang County

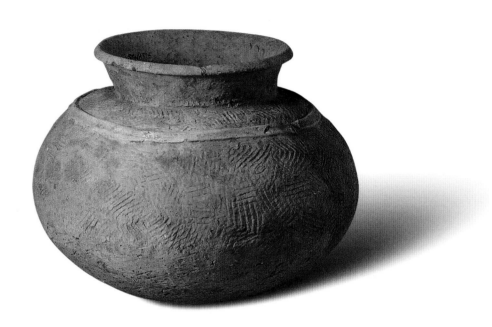

硬陶罐

马桥文化

陶质

口径 11 厘米，高 14 厘米

1997 年浙江遂昌好川墓地出土。

遂昌县文物管理委员会藏

Hard Pottery Jar

Maqiao Culture

Pottery

Mouth Diameter 11 cm/ Height 14 cm

The jar was excavated from Haochuan Cemetery at Suichang County, Zhejiang Province.

Preserved in Department of Cultural Relics Coneservation of Suichang County

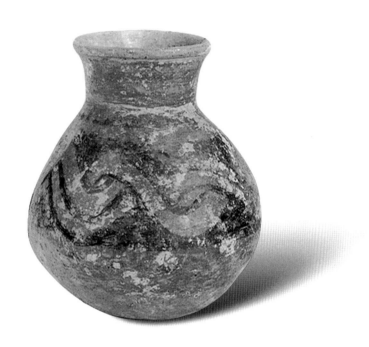

彩陶罐

石家河文化

陶质

通高 13.2 厘米

荆州博物馆藏

Painted Pottery Jar

Shijiahe Culture

Pottery

Height 13.2 cm

Preserved in Jingzhou Museum

新石器时代晚期，大汶口文化北庄一期 (前 4000—前 3500)

红陶质

口径 7 厘米，底径 5 厘米，高 27 厘米

Small-mouthed Red Pottery Jar

First Phase of Beizhuang Sites of Dawenkou Culture (4000 B.C.–3500 B.C.), Late Neolithic Age

Red Pottery

Mouth Diameter 7 cm/ Bottom Diameter 5 cm/ Height 27 cm

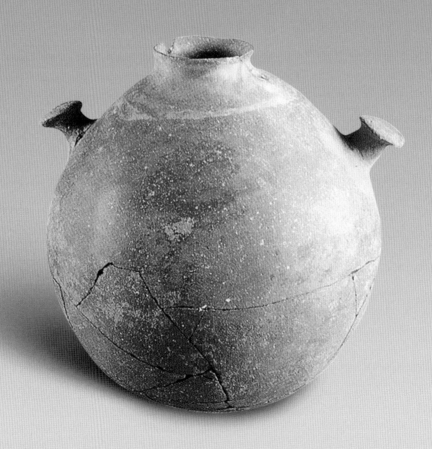

器表通施红色陶衣。汲水及存水的器具，有时也用于煮食。此件约为个人外出所携带的用具，两侧的蘑菇状把手便于携带背挎，小口可防止行进中水或食物外溅。山东省长岛县北庄遗址出土。

北京大学赛克勒考古与艺术博物馆藏

The vessel is covered entirely with red coating. It was utilized for storing and drawing water, or cooking food occasionally. The jar is a food or water carrying device, comprising easy-to-carry mushroom-shaped handles at both sides and a small mouth for preventing the splash of food or water. It was unearthed from the Site of Beizhuang at Changdao County, Shandong Province.

Preserved in Arthur M. Sackler Museum of Art and Archaeology at Peking University

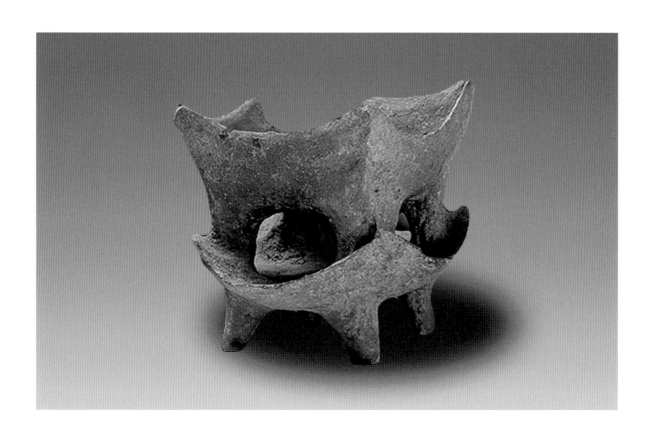

四足双层陶方鼎

新石器时代

夹砂陶质

通高 13 厘米

Double-decker Quadripod "Ding" with Four Legs

Neolithic Age

Sandy Pottery

Height 13 cm

该鼎由上下二层组成，手工捏制，外表施橘红装饰土。一层底部四足锥足外撇，器腹较浅，口沿垂弧，内壁及二层外底部留有使用过的痕迹。二层的足与底层翘角处连接，直腹，内底方而平，口沿弧形，四角高于口部，造型古拙别致，线条自然流畅，为出土器物中罕见，推测可能是原始先民保存火种的用器。

高淳区文物保管所藏

The "Ding" (Pot) was kneaded by hand into double layers and was coated with orange engobe. There are four cone feet turning outside under the base of the lower deck, above which is a relatively shallow abdomen and a sagging rim. Clear signs of use can be seen on the interior wall and the bottom of the upper deck, whose feet are connected to the rake angles of the lower deck. With straight abdomen, squared and flat inner bottom, curved rim and four angles exceeding the mouth, the upper deck is made in an unsophisticated but unique style with natural and smooth lines. This design is rare among the objects unearthed. It is presumed that this appliance was used by the primitive residents for keeping the fire.

Preserved in Cultural Relics Preservation of Gaochun District

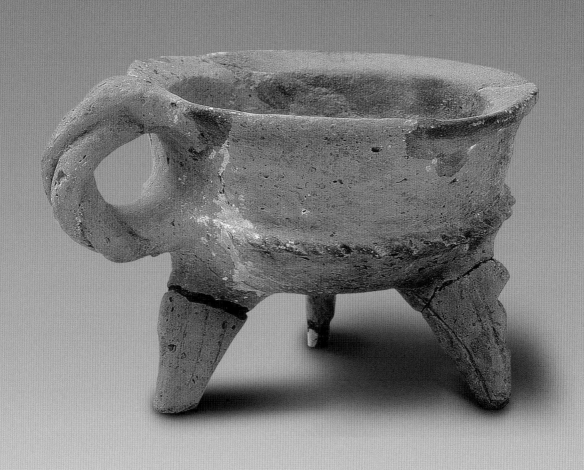

带把陶鼎

新石器时代

陶质

口径 10 厘米，通高 8.2 厘米

红陶，口微侈，腹中部饰一周绚索状堆纹，腹侧有一扭索形把手。窄面向外的三角形扁足，

足边缘压成锯齿状，两侧有平竖划纹。江苏南京北阴阳营遗址 247 号墓出土。

南京博物院藏

Handled Pottery "Ding" (Tripod)

Neolithic Age

Pottery

Mouth Diameter 10 cm/ Height 8.2 cm

The red pottery "Ding" (tripod) has a slightly flared mouth. The middle of the abdomen is adorned with a band of raised stripes of rope veins. A handle in the shape of a twisted rope is attached to the side of the abdomen. With the narrow end facing outward, the triangular oblate feet are engrailed on the fringe and are decorated with smooth vertical lines at both sides. It was excavated from No. 247 Tomb of Beiyinyangying Site in Nanjing, Jiangsu Province.

Preserved in Nanjing Museum

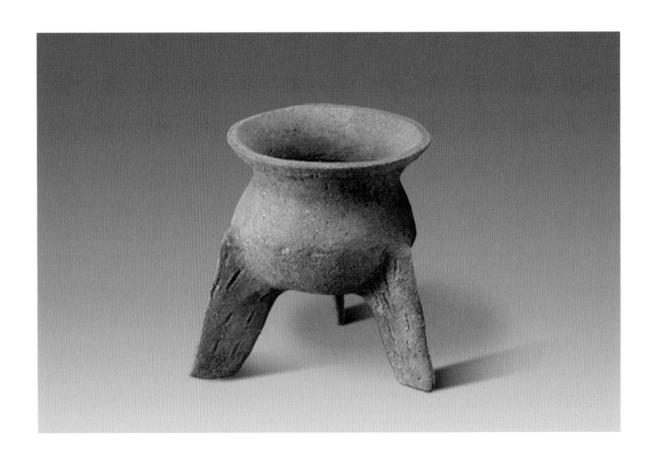

陶鼎

良渚文化

陶质

口径 12.8 厘米，高 16 厘米

Pottery "Ding" (Tripod)

Liangzhu Culture

Pottery

Mouth Diameter 12.8 cm/ Height 16 cm

夹砂红陶。敞口，束颈，折腹，鱼鳍足，腹
中部饰一周凸棱。1988 年余杭良渚庙前遗址
出土。

浙江省文物考古研究所藏

This pottery "Ding" (tripod) is made of red
sandy pottery. It features a flared mouth, a
contracted neck, an angular abdomen and fin-
shaped feet. A raised band of ridge is found
around the middle of the abdomen. It was
excavated from the Miaoqian Site of the Liangzhu
Culture at Yuhang District in the year 1988.
Preserved in Institute of Cultural Relics and
Archaeology of Zhejiang Province

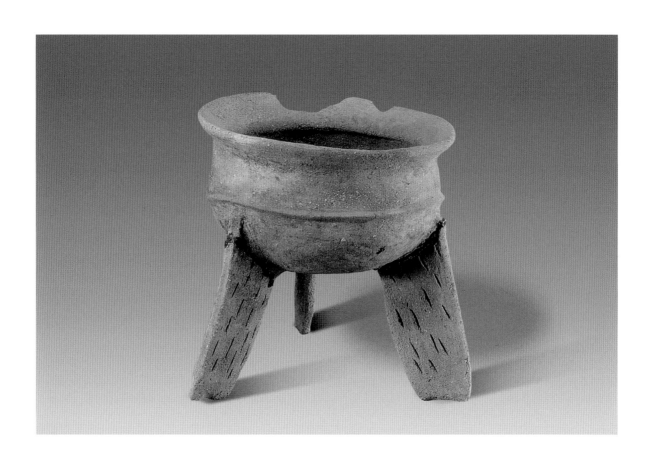

陶鼎

良渚文化

陶质

口径 8 厘米，高 16.8 厘米

Pottery "Ding" (Tripod)

Liangzhu Culture

Pottery

Mouth Diameter 8 cm/ Height 16.8 cm

夹砂红陶。敞口，束颈，折腹，鱼鳍足，腹中部饰一周凸棱。1988 年余杭良渚庙前遗址出土。

浙江省文物考古研究所藏

This pottery "Ding" (tripod) is made of red sandy pottery. It features a flared mouth, a contracted neck, an angular abdomen and fin-shaped feet. A raised band of ridge is found around the middle of the abdomen. It was excavated from the Miaoqian Site of the Liangzhu Culture at Yuhang District in the year 1988.

Preserved in Institute of Cultural Relics and Archaeology of Zhejiang Province

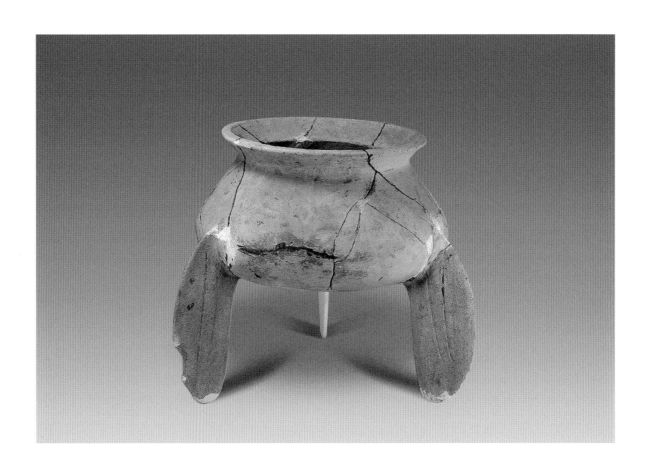

陶鼎

良渚文化

陶质

口径 25.5 厘米，高 33 厘米

Pottery "Ding" (Tripod)

Liangzhu Culture

Pottery

Mouth Diameter 25.5 cm/ Height 33 cm

夹砂灰红陶。敞口平唇，缩颈溜肩，圜底较平缓，侧面鱼鳍形三鼎足，足两侧划有三道竖向直线。造型规整，为实用炊器。

浙江省文物考古研究所藏

The "Ding" (tripod) is made of grayish-red sandy pottery. It has a flared mouth, a flat mouth rim, a contracted neck, a sloping shoulder and a gently curved round bottom. There are three fin-shaped feet attached to the bottom side, on the flank of which are carved three vertical lines. The regular shaped vessel was utilized as a daily cooking utensil.

Preserved in Institute of Cultural Relics and Archaeology of Zhejiang Province

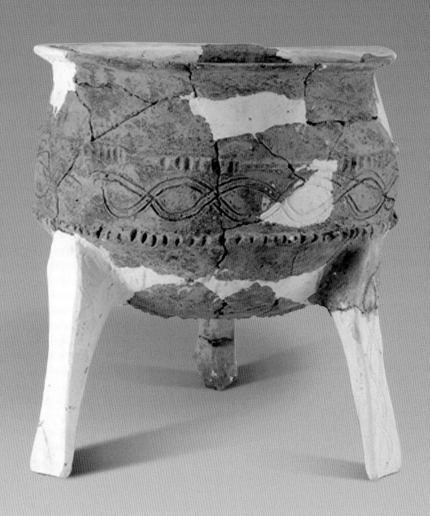

陶鼎

崧泽文化晚期良渚文化早期

陶质

口径 24 厘米，高 26.2 厘米

粗泥陶，胎多孔隙。深釜形腹，器内腹底转折处设置箅隔，圜底，凿形足。器腹中段饰绞索状刻划纹和压印窝点的突棱组合纹饰，三足外侧也饰索状刻划纹，器底饰三叉形压印窝点的突脊。

海盐县博物馆藏

Pottery "Ding" (Tripod)

Late Songze Culture/ Early Liangzhu Culture

Pottery

Mouth Diameter 24 cm/ Height 26.2 cm

This pottery "Ding" was made of coarse clay, with a lot of small openings on the body. The abdomen is in the shape of a deep cauldron. At the flexure of the inner bottom is set a grate. The "Ding" has a round bottom and scalpriform feet. The middle part of the abdomen is decorated with carved noose patterns combined with raised ridges stamped with pores. The lateral borders of the tri-foot are incised with noose patterns too. The bottom of the pot is decorated with raised ridges in trident shape with stamped pores.

Preserved in Haiyan Museum

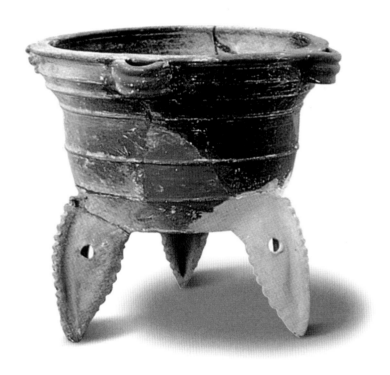

夹砂灰陶鸟足鼎

新石器时代晚期，山东龙山文化 (前 2500—前 2000)

陶质

口径 18.5 厘米，底径 10 厘米，高 16 厘米

Grey Sandy Pottery "Ding" (Tripod) with Bird Legs

Longshan Culture of Shandong Province (2500 B.C. – 2000 B.C.), Late Neolithic Age

Pottery

Mouth Diameter 18.5 cm/ Bottom Diameter 10 cm/ Height 16 cm

该藏黑色的外观、轮制的工艺及鸟形的装饰，

无一不体现了山东龙山文化特有的风格。炊

具。山东省潍坊市姚官庄遗址出土。

北京大学赛克勒考古与艺术博物馆藏

The dark appearance, the wheel-thrown craftmanship and the decoration of a bird design of this "Ding" (tripod) all represent the unique style of the Longshan Culture in Shandong Province. It was used as a cooking vessel. It was excavated from the Yaoguanzhuang Site of Weifang City, Shandong Province.

Preserved in Arthur M. Sackler Museum of Art and Archaeology at Peking University

黑陶鸟头形足鼎

新石器时代，龙山文化

黑陶质

口径 26 厘米，高 18.3 厘米

Black Pottery "Ding" (Tripod) with Bird-Head Feet

Longshan Culture, Neolithic Age

Black Pottery

Mouth Diameter 26 cm/ Height 18.3 cm

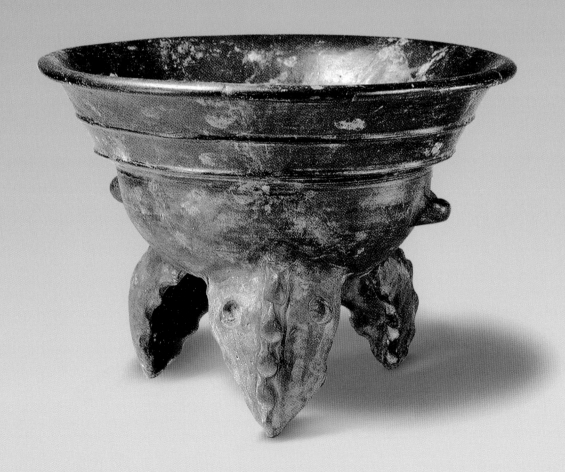

胎中夹细砂，施黑陶衣，器表漆黑发亮。器身作盆形，大敞口，口沿外卷，折腹，平底，下附三个鸟头形足。足呈等腰三角形，上部宽而下部尖圆，足面上鼓下凹，中央饰堆纹，两侧有眼眶，足下部向内弯呈鸟嘴形。鸟头作为陶器上的装饰题材，与东夷族以鸟为图腾有关，鸟头形足鼎又是黄河下游龙山文化典型器物。1960 年潍坊市姚官庄出土。

山东博物馆藏

The body of this pottery "Ding" (tripod) is mixed with fine sand. The whole vessel is coated with shiny black glaze. The basin-shaped vessel has a big flared mouth, an everted rim, an angular abdomen and a flat bottom, to which are attached three feet in the shape of bird heads. The foot is shaped into an isosceles triangle, with a wide top tapering down to a pointed round underpart. The surface of the feet is convex at the top and concave at the bottom, the central area of which is decorated with raised stripes. Bird's eyes are found on both sides of the stripes. The lower part of the foot is bending inwards as a beak. The bird head is used as decoration for pottery ware due to the bird totem of the Eastern Yi nationality. "Ding" with bird-head feet is typical of the Longshan culture in the downstream areas of the Yellow River. It was excavated from Yaoguanzhuang Site of Weifang City in the year 1960.

Preserved in Shandong Museum

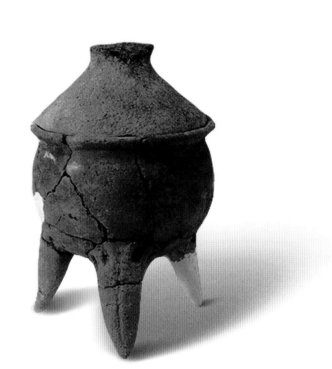

带盖陶鼎

河姆渡文化三期

陶质

口径 14 厘米，通高 16.6 厘米

盖：口径 13.2 厘米，高 6.4 厘米

1990 年象山县塔山遗址出土。

象山县文物管理委员会藏

Pottery Tripod "Ding" (Tripod) with Lid

Hemudu Culture Ⅲ

Pottery

Mouth Diameter 14 cm/ Height 16.6 cm

Lid: Mouth Diameter 13.2 cm/ Height 6.4 cm

This tripod "Ding" was excavated from the Tashan Archaeological Site in Xiangshan County, Zhejiang Province, in the year 1990.

Preserved in Xiangshan County Administration Committee of Cultural Relics

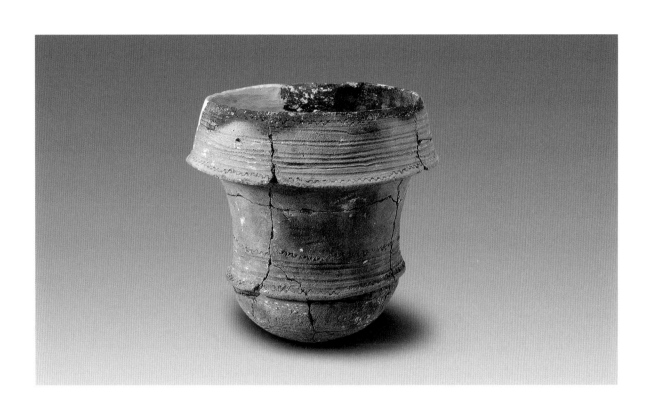

陶釜

河姆渡文化

陶质

口径 18 厘米，高 19 厘米

夹炭陶，敛口，肩脊，口沿和肩脊处饰蚶壳刺印纹。

浙江省文物考古研究所藏

Pottery "Fu" (Cauldron)

Hemudu Culture

Pottery

Mouth Diameter 18 cm/ Height 19 cm

This charcoal-mixed pottery "Fu" (cauldron) has a contracted mouth and a shoulder ridge. Both the mouth rim and the shoulder ridge are adorned with impressed designs of cockle shell thorn.

Preserved in Institute of Cultural Relics and Archaeology of Zhejiang Province

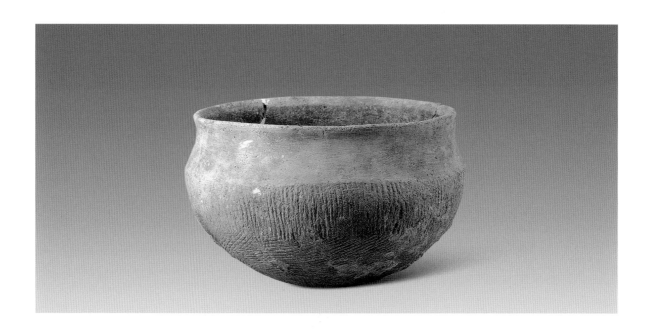

陶釜

河姆渡文化

陶质

口径 22.5 厘米，高 15 厘米

1996 年余姚市鯔山遗址出土。

浙江省文物考古研究所藏

Pottery "Fu" (Cauldron)

Hemudu Culture

Pottery

Mouth Diameter 22.5 cm/ Height 15 cm

The cauldron was excavated at the Archaeological Site of Zishan in Yuyao City in the year 1996.

Preserved in Institute of Cultural Relics and Archaeology of Zhejiang Province

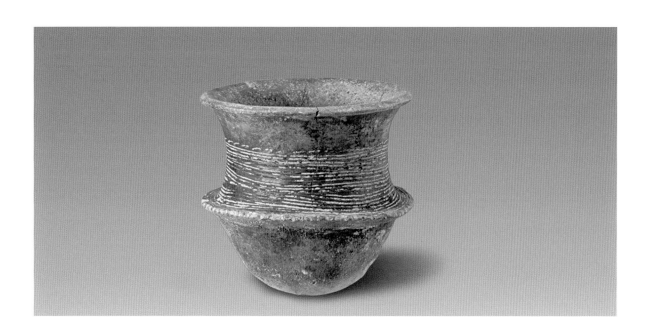

陶釜

河姆渡文化

陶质

口径 21.6 厘米，高 20 厘米

1996 年余姚市鲻山遗址出土。

浙江省文物考古研究所藏

Pottery "Fu" (Cauldron)

Hemudu Culture

Pottery

Mouth Diameter 21.6 cm/ Height 20 cm

The cauldron was excavated at the archaeological Site of Zishan in Yuyao City in the year 1996.

Preserved in Institute of Cultural Relics and Archaeology of Zhejiang Province

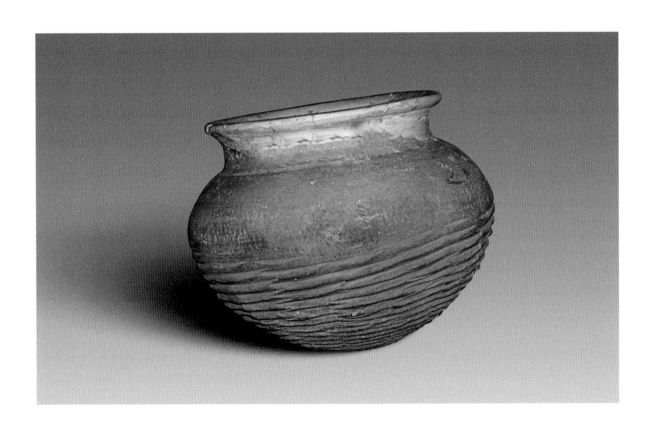

陶釜

新石器时代

陶质

口径 14.2 厘米，通高 14 厘米，重 800 克

Pottery "Fu" (Cauldron)

Neolithic Age

Pottery

Mouth Diameter 14.2 cm/ Height 14 cm/ Weight 800 g

圆唇，鼓腹，圜底，腹下筐纹。夹砂红陶。炊器。

口沿有修补。陕西省西安市征集。

陕西医史博物馆藏

This pottery "Fu" (cauldron) features a round
rim, a swelling belly and a round-arc-bottom.
The lower abdomen adorned with basket weave
patterns is made of red pottery mixed with sand.
The cauldron with the mouth rim restored was
used as a cooking utensil. It was collected from
Xi'an, Shaanxi Province.

Preserved in Shaanxi Museum of Medical History

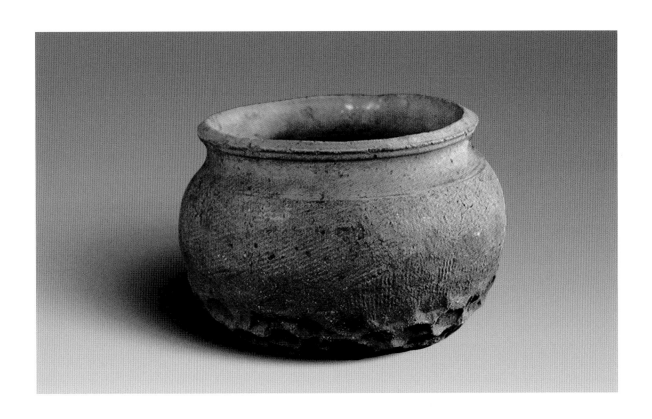

陶釜

新石器时代

夹砂红陶质

口径 19.5 厘米，通高 15.5 厘米，重 2200 克

Pottery "Fu" (Cauldron)

Neolithic Age

Red Sandy Pottery

Mouth Diameter 19.5 cm/ Height 15.5 cm/ Weight 2,200 g

侈口，圆腹，圈底。腹为绳纹，底为石头纹。生活用器具，炊具。完整无损。陕西省渭南市征集。

陕西医史博物馆藏

This pottery "Fu" (cauldron) has a flared mouth, a swelling belly decorated with cord pattern and a circular bottom adorned with rock stripes. The cauldron, well-kept, was used as a household utensil and cooking vessel. It was collected in Weinan City, Shaanxi Province.

Preserved in Shaanxi Museum of Medical History

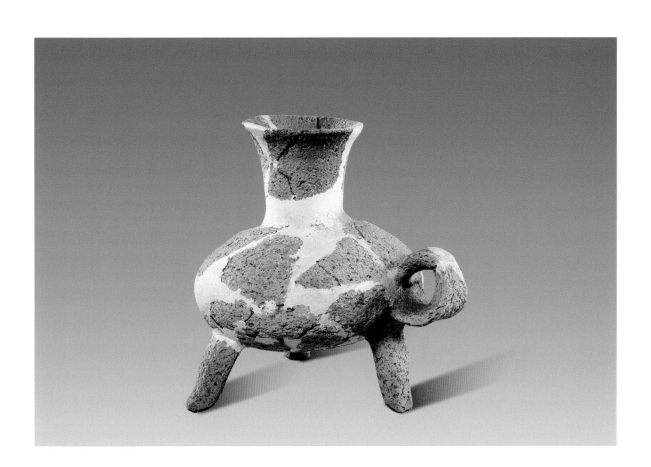

陶釜

新石器时代，崧泽文化

夹砂红陶质

高 17 厘米

Pottery "Fu" (Cauldron)

Songze Culture, Neolithic Age

Red Sandy Pottery

Height 17 cm

侈口，高领，扁球腹，三个扁凿形实足，足
尖外撇。器物比例匀称。

常州博物馆藏

This pottery "Fu" (cauldron) is designed with a
flared mouth, a high collar, an oblate spheroid
shaped belly and three flat chisel-shaped solid
legs with flaring toes. The vessel is well-
proportioned.

Preserved in Changzhou Museum

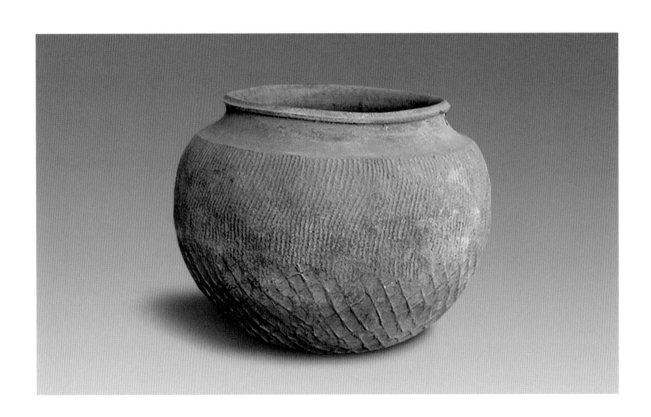

红陶釜

新石器时代

陶质

口径 21.5 厘米，腹围 97 厘米，高 25 厘米，重 3350 克

Red Pottery "Fu" (Cauldron)

Neolithic Age

Pottery

Mouth Diameter 21.5 cm/ Belly Perimeter 97 cm/ Height 25 cm/ Weight 3,350 g

圆唇，折肩，圆腹底，肩部有一印记。腹上部为绳纹，腹底部为菱形纹。炊器。完整无损。陕西省澄城县征集。

陕西医史博物馆藏

With a round rim, an angular shoulder and a round-arc-bottom, this "Fu" (cauldron) bears a mark on the shoulder. The upper part of the belly is decorated with cord patterns and the lower part is adorned with lozenge patterns. The cauldron served as a cooking utensil, and it remains intact. It was collected from Chengcheng County, Shaanxi Province.

Preserved in Shaanxi Museum of Medical History

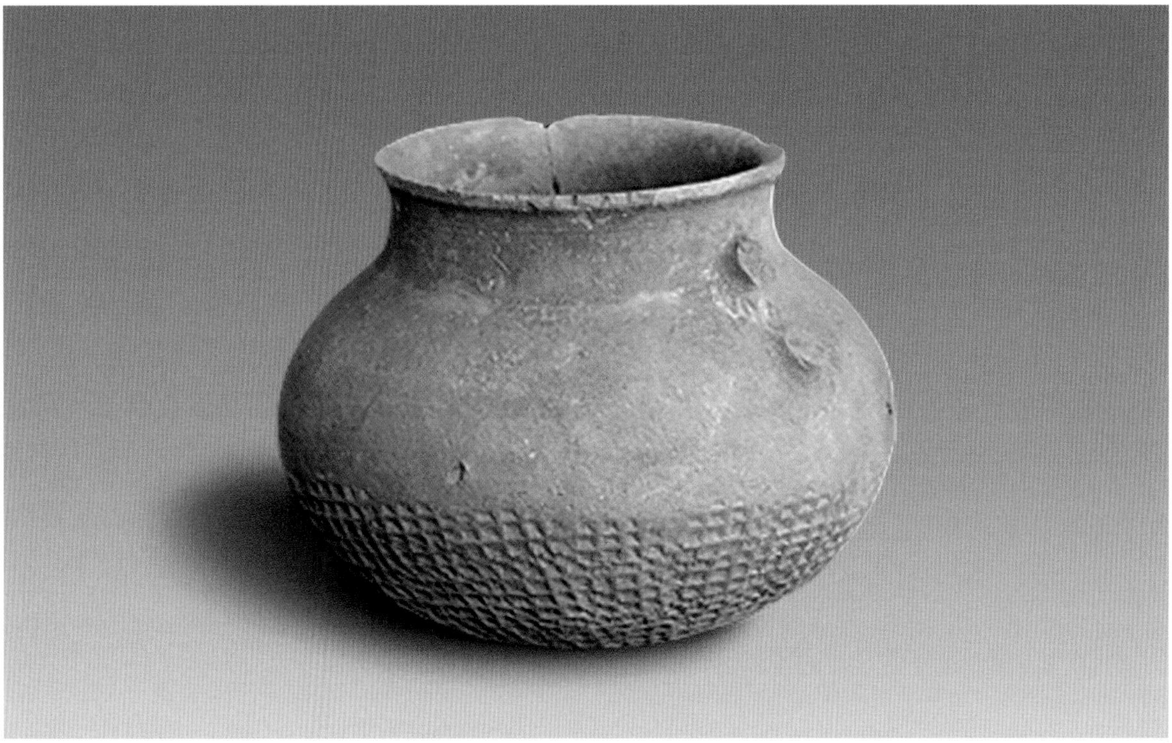

单耳红陶釜

新石器时代

红陶质

口径 8 厘米，高 9.5 厘米，重 250 克

Red Pottery "Fu" (Cauldron) with Single Ear

Neolithic Age

Red Pottery

Mouth Diameter 8 cm/ Height 9.5 cm/ Weight 250 g

侈口，溜肩，圆腹，圜底。底部为筐纹，肩
部有一印记。炊器。口沿略残，肩部有一耳残。
陕西省白水县杨家沟征集。

陕西医史博物馆藏

This red pottery "Fu" (cauldron) features
a flared mouth, a sloping shoulder, a round
abdomen and a round-arcbottom. On the
shoulder is set one single ear. The bottom
is adorned with basket weave patterns. The
shoulder bears a mark. This cauldron, with
the mouth rim and ear cracked, was used
as a cooking utensil. It was collected from
Yangjiagou Village, Baishui County, Shaanxi
Province.

Preserved in Shaanxi Museum of Medical History

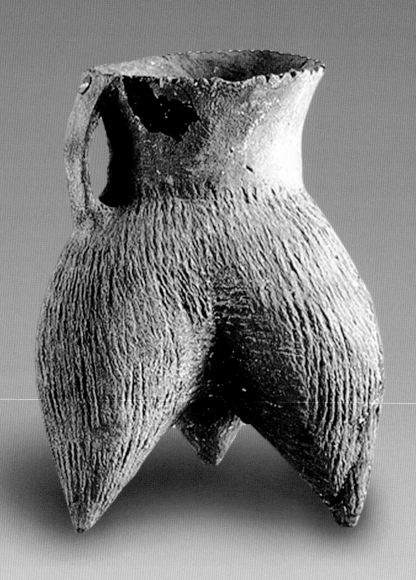

灰陶单耳鬲

新石器时代晚期，客省庄文化 (前 2600—前 2000)

灰陶质

口径 12.5 厘米，高 23.3 厘米

新石器时代晚期主要的炊器。鬲的外形似鼎，但三足内空，目的是为了增大受热面积以更好地利用热能。它的主要用途是煮粥、制羹和烧水，与甑、甗类蒸食器有所不同。胎料中加有大量的粗砂，其造型与装饰具有强烈的地域风格。陕西省西安市长安区阿底村出土。

北京大学赛克勒考古与艺术博物馆藏

Grey Pottery "Li" (Cauldron) with Single Ear

Keshengzhuang Culture (2600 B.C.－2000 B.C.) , Late Neolithic Age

Grey Pottery

Mouth Diameter 12.5 cm/ Height 23.3 cm

"Li" (Cauldron) is a primary cooking utensil in the late period of the Neolithic age. This object with three hollow pouch-like legs resembles an ancient tripod. The primary function of these legs is to increase the total surface area exposed to the heat of the fire, and thereby speed up the cooking process. Different from steamers such as "Zeng" and "Yen", "Li" is mainly used for cooking rice congee, boiling soup and heating water. The roughcast is mixed with a lot of coarse sand. Its design and decorations have a strong regional flavor. It was excavated from Adi Village in Chang'an District, Xi'an City, Shaanxi Province.

Preserved in Arthur M. Sackler Museum of Art and Archaeology at Peking University

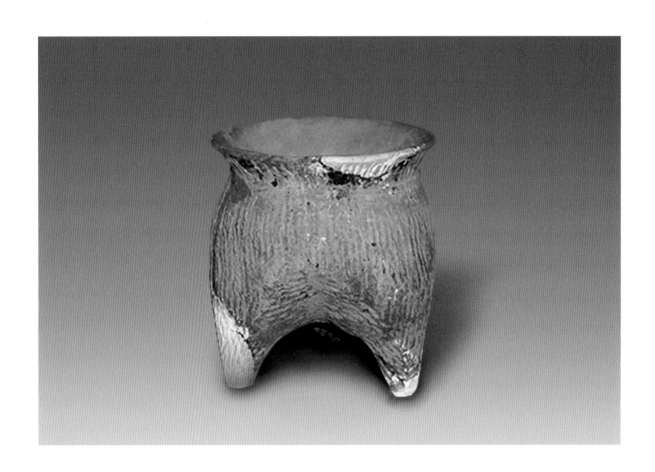

陶鬲

新石器时代

灰陶质

口径 12.8 厘米，通高 13.5 厘米，重 580 克

Pottery "Li" (Cauldron)

Neolithic Age

Grey Pottery

Mouth Diameter 12.8 cm/ Height 13.5 cm/ Weight 580 g

侈口，三乳足，周身粗绳纹。口沿、两足有
修补。炊器。陕西省乾县征集。

陕西医史博物馆藏

This pottery cauldron features a flared mouth,
three nipple-like feet and a grey body. It is
covered entirely with thick cord patterns.
The mouth rim and two of the feet have been
restored. The cauldron served as a cooking
utensil. It was collected from Qianxian County,
Shaanxi Province.

Preserved in Shaanxi Museum of Medical History

夹砂灰陶绳纹鬲

新石器时代晚期，河南龙山文化 (前 2600—前 2000)

陶质

口径 28 ～ 29 厘米，高 52.2 厘米

Grey Sandy Pottery "Li" (Cauldron) with Cord Patterns

Longshan Culture of Henan Province (2600 B.C.–2000 B.C.) , Late Neolithic Age

Pottery

Mouth Diameter 28–29 cm/ Height 52.2 cm

从该藏上、下分离明显及功能多样两方面观察，这种鬲在造型与用途上都介于普通炊鬲和炊甗之间。此鬲综合采用模制、轮制、手制多种制陶工艺，以夹砂陶制成，陶胎厚重，陶色纯正，形制巨大，实为近年出土的龙山炊具中的精品。河南省济源市原城遗址出土。

河南省文物考古研究院藏

With a clear division of the upper and lower section and its diverse functions, this pottery "Li" (cauldron) is similar to both ordinary cauldrons and steamers in shape and function. It was made with a variety of pottery making techniques, such as moulding, wheel-making and hand-making. This large pottery "Li", made of sand-embedded pottery with a pure colour, is regarded as an exquisite example of the cooking utensils excavated from Longshan in recent years. It was unearthed from the Yuancheng Site in Jiyuan City, Henan Province.
Preserved in Henan Provincial Institute of Cultural Heritage and Archaeology

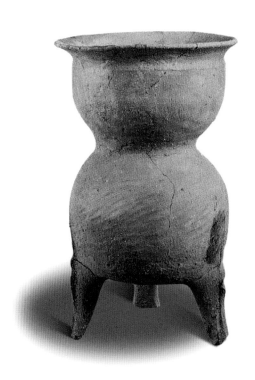

夹砂红陶甗

新石器时代，大汶口文化晚期 (前 2800—前 2500)

夹砂红陶质

口径 16.5 厘米，高 27.7 厘米

Red Sandy Pottery "Yan" (Steamer)

Neolithic Age, Late Period of Dawenkou Culture (2800 B.C. –2500 B.C.)

Red Sandy Pottery

Mouth Diameter 16.5 cm/ Height 27.7 cm

造型稳重。上古时期的复合烹饪器，即具无底的甑和无耳空足的鬲的复合结构，实际上就是一套蒸锅，并兼具灶和锅的双重功能。汉以后甗作为炊具逐渐被淘汰。山东诸城市前寨遗址出土。

北京大学赛克勒考古与艺术博物馆藏

This "Yan" (steamer) is a compound set of cooking utensils with a steady shape in ancient times. It comprises a steamer Zeng with no bottom and a hollow-legged cauldron "Li" with no ears. It is in fact a steamer set with dual functions of both an oven and a pot. The steamer "Yan" used as a cooking utensil fell into disuse gradually after the Han Dynasty. It was excavated from the Qianzhai Site, Zhucheng City, Shandong Province.

Preserved in Arthur M. Sackler Museum of Art and Archaeology at Peking University

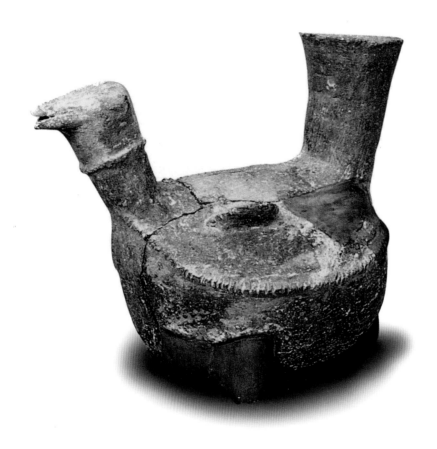

灰陶鸟形鬶

新石器时代晚期，大汶口文化北庄一期 (前 4000—前 3500)

灰陶质

长 23.5 厘米，高 19 厘米

Bird-shaped Grey Pottery "Gui" (Vessel)

First Phase of Beizhuang Sites of Dawenkou Culture (4000 B.C.–3500 B.C.), Late Neolithic Age

Grey Pottery

Length 23.5 cm/ Height 19 cm

鬶的功用与鬲相同，也是烹煮食品的器具，但因它具有尖嘴（即"流"）和把手（即"鋬"），所以它无须借助于勺而可以直接将煮好的食品倒入食具且不致溅溢，因而在功能上较鬲先进。山东省长岛县北庄遗址出土。

北京大学赛克勒考古与艺术博物馆藏

Pottery "Gui" (vessel) has the same function as pottery tripod "Li". Both are cooking utensils. Bearing a spout and a handle, the Gui can be held easily to pour out the boiled food to tableware without spilling it. "Gui" is more advanced in function than pottery tripod "Li". It was excavated from the Beizhuang Site of Changdao County in Shandong Province. Preserved in Arthur M. Sackler Museum of Art and Archaeology at Peking University

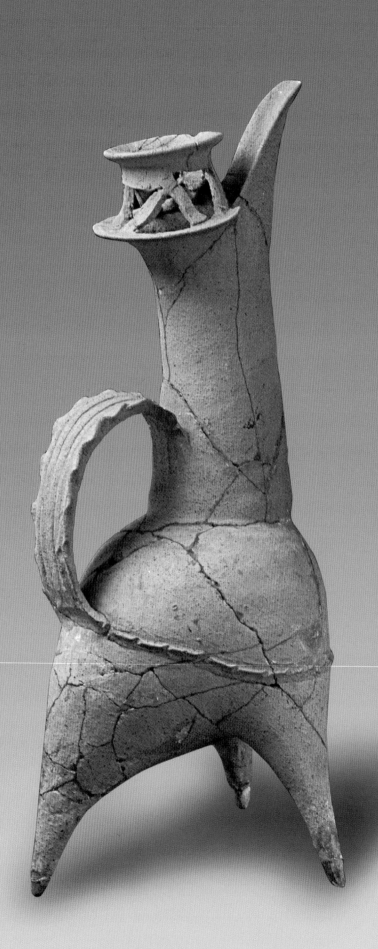

白陶双层口鬶

新石器时代，大汶口文化

夹砂白陶

高 36.8 厘米

手工塑制。鸟喙形流上昂，细颈高直，宽肥腹，空足高尖，宽带式鋬。双层口沿，中间饰三角形镂孔。双层口式陶鬶极为罕见，既可阻挡灰尘杂物入内，又富有很强的装饰效果。1978 年临沂市大范庄出土。

临沂市博物馆藏

White Pottery "Gui" (Wine Vessel) with a Double-deck Mouth

Dawenkou Culture, Neolithic Age

White Sandy Pottery

Height 36.8 cm

Moulded manually, this pottery "Gui" (wine vessel) has a beak-shaped spout stretching upward, a thin and straight high neck, a wide and fat abdomen, three hollow legs with high heels, and a handle in the form of a wide belt. A double-deck mouth is adorned with openwork designs of triangles in between the decks. This pottery "Gui" (wine vessel) with a double-deck mouth is extremely rare. This type of mouth can not only keep dirt out but also renders a strong decorative effect. It was excavated from Dafanzhuang Village in Linyi City in the year 1978.

Preserved in Linyi Museum

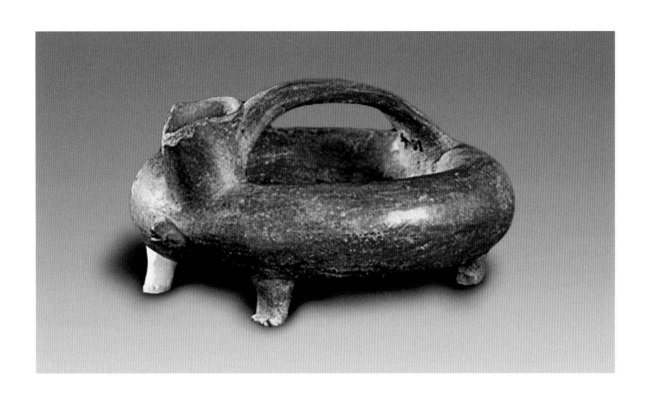

红陶龟形鬶

新石器时代，大汶口文化

红陶质

长 20.5 厘米，宽 19 厘米，高 10.5 厘米

Turtle-shaped Red Pottery "Gui" (Wine Vessel)

Dawenkou Culture, Neolithic Age

Red Pottery

Length 20.5 cm/ Width 19 cm/ Height 10.5 cm

红色陶土中夹杂有云母片，手工捏塑，通体
施红陶衣，压磨光滑。器作圆龟形，头上有流，
腹呈圆筒形，下附四足，上安提手。题材新颖，
制作精巧，既是盛水（或酒）容器，又是原
始陶塑艺术品。1979年山东省胶州市三里
河出土。

胶州市博物馆藏

This wine vessel "Gui" (wine vessel) is made
of red pottery mixed with mica sheets and
moulded by hands. The whole vessel is covered
with smooth red coating through pressing
and grinding. Round in shape like a turtle, the
vessel has a spout as the head and a cylinder-
shaped abdomen. It rests atop four short legs
and has a handle attached to the upper part
of the abdomen. With a novel design and
exquisite workmanship, this pottery Gui is
not only a common water and wine container,
but a primitive pottery work of art as well. It
was excavated from Sanlihe in Jiaozhou City,
Shandong Province.

Preserved in Jiaozhou Museum

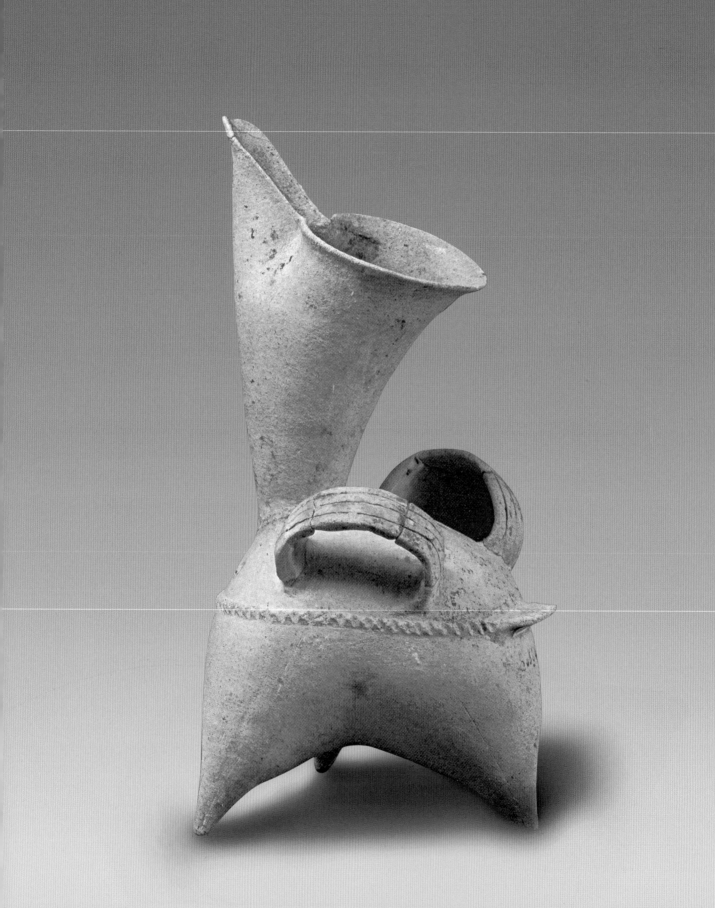

白陶双鋬鬶

新石器时代，大汶口文化

夹砂白陶

高 34.1 厘米

手工塑制。鸟喙形流上昂，颈细而高，腹部微鼓，三袋足。背部安双宽带式鋬，后部翘起尾形堡，堡上刻画菱纹。形象如鸟，展翅欲飞。传说东夷族以禽鸟为其图腾，故塑造出似鸟形的各式陶器，成为富有地方文化特点的器物。

莒州博物馆藏

White Pottery "Gui" (Wine Vessel) with Two Handles

Dawenkou Culture, Neolithic Age

White Sandy Pottery

Height 34.1 cm

This pottery "Gui" (wine vessel) is moulded manually with features of a beak-shaped spout stretching upward, a high slim neck, a slightly swelling abdomen and three pouched feet. On the back are two wide belt-shaped handles with socket patterns, and to the rear is attached an upwarp tail with carved designs. The design of this pottery "Gui" (wine vessel) looks like a bird, ready to spread its wings to fly. Legend says that the Eastern barbarians at that time regarded birds as their totem, so they designed various pottery vessels in the shape of birds with strong regional cultural characteristics.

Preserved in Juzhou Museum

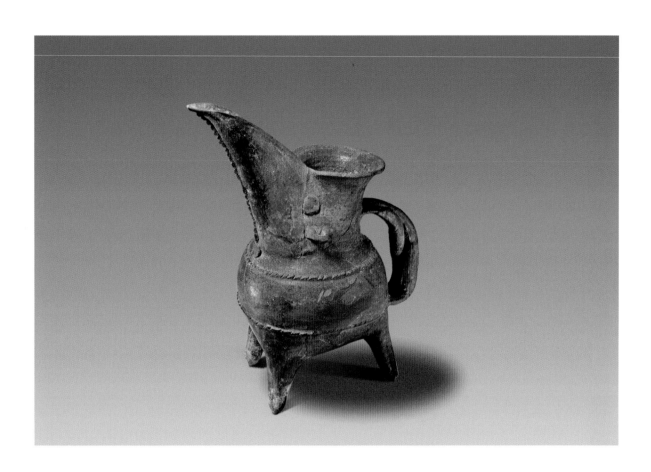

红陶实足鬶

新石器时代，龙山文化

夹砂红陶

通高 32.4 厘米

Red Pottery "Gui" (Wine Vessel) with Solid Feet

Longshan Culture, Neolithic Age

Red Sandy Pottery

Height 32.4 cm

手工塑制，施棕红色陶衣，压磨光滑。鸟喙形长流高高上仰，侈口短颈，圆腹平裆，锥形实足，双股竖鋬。流下及腹部饰有锯齿状附加堆纹，颈两侧有耳和圆饼，象征禽鸟的双耳与双眼。形象生动，制作精湛，既是实用水器皿，又是富有地方文化特色的陶塑艺术品。1960年山东省潍坊市姚官庄出土。

山东博物馆藏

This pottery "Gui" (wine vessel) is moulded manually and covered with smooth brownish red coating through pressing and grinding. With a beak-shaped spout highly stretching upward, the vessel has a flared mouth, a short neck, a round abdomen which is ventrally flattened, three cone-shaped solid feet and vertical handles made of two strands of clay. Two raised zigzag stripes are found under the spout and on the abdomen. On both sides of the neck are set ears and small round spots, resembling a bird's ears and eyes. With a vivid design and exquisite workmanship, it is not only a functional water vessel, but also a pottery work of art with strong regional cultural characteristics. It was excavated from Yaoguanzhuang Site in Weifang City, Shandong Province, in the year 1960.

Preserved in Shandong Museum

新石器时代晚期，山东龙山文化 (前 2500—
前 2000)

红陶质

口径 20.4 厘米，高 36.8 厘米

Longshan Culture, Shandong Province (2500 B.C. -
2000 B.C), Late Neolithic Age

Red Pottery

Mouth Diameter 20.4 cm/ Height 36.8 cm

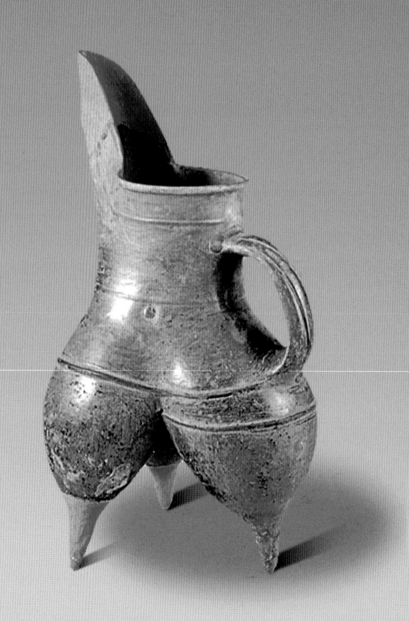

红色胎体，但成型后外表经过磨光工艺，使器
身光润亮泽而呈灰黄色，避免了在不施彩情况
下外观的粗糙。造型极富神韵，装饰洗练。煮
食的炊具。山东省日照市两城镇遗址出土。

　　北京大学赛克勒考古与艺术博物馆藏

This pottery "Gui" (wine vessel) has a red rough
casting. After forming, the vessel surface was
burnished and appeared smooth and glossy
in greyish yellow, rather than the roughness
of unglazed appearance. The design is rich in
romantic charm with the decoration simple and
unsophisticated. The vessel served as a cooking
utensil. It was excavated at the archaeological
Site of Liangcheng Town, Rizhao City, Shandong
Province.
Preserved in Arthur M. Sackler Museum of Art
and Archaeology at Peking University

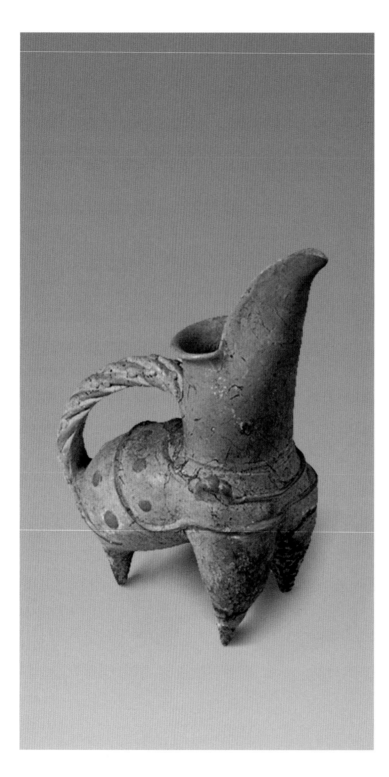

橙黄陶袋足鬶

新石器时代，龙山文化

橙黄陶质

通高 29.2 厘米

Orange Pottery "Gui" (Wine Vessel) with Pouched Feet

Longshan Culture, Neolithic Age

Orange Pottery

Height 29.2 cm

胎中夹砂，手工塑制，压磨光滑，施有陶衣，器表为橙黄色。鸟喙形流向上斜伸，侈口卷沿，直筒形颈。三袋足分裆而立，前两足作对称状，后足肥大且向后伸，三足位置呈等腰三角形。扭绳式錾跨颈与后足间。颈下两侧饰附耳，袋足上饰曲线状附加堆纹，遍身贴附小圆饼饰。整器犹如一只珍禽瑞鸟昂首而立，实属罕见的陶塑艺术品。1960 年山东省潍坊市姚官庄出土。

山东博物馆藏

This sandy pottery "Gui" (wine vessel) is moulded manually and covered with smooth orange coating through pressing and grinding. With a beak-shaped spout obliquely upward, this vessel has a flared mouth, a rolled rim, a cylindrical neck and three pouched feet standing separately. Two symmetrical front feet and a plump rear foot form an isosceles triangle. A twisted rope-shaped handle is set between the neck and the rear feet. Rings are found under the neck. The punched feet are adorned with curved raised stripes, and the whole body is decorated with small round spots. Like an exotic bird standing steadfast with head held high, this vessel is indeed a rare pottery work of art. It was excavated from Yaoguanzhuang Site in Weifang City, Shandong Province, in the year 1960.

Preserved in Shandong Museum

陶鬶

马桥文化

陶质

高 24.6 厘米

遂昌县文物管理委员会藏

Pottery "Gui" (Wine Vessel)

Maqiao Culture

Pottery

Height 24.6 cm

Preserved in Department of Cultural Relics

Coneservation of Suichang County

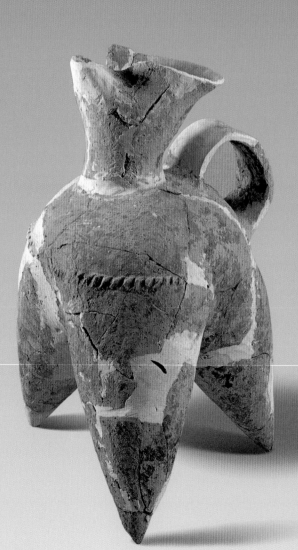

彩陶缶

新石器时代（马厂类型）

陶质

口径 19 厘米，高 33.4 厘米

唇微侈，鼓腹，腹双耳，正面浮雕人头像，

下为浮塑彩绘人体，背为蛙纹，两侧网纹。

青海柳湾六坪台出土。

青海柳湾彩陶博物馆藏

Pot with Naked Human Figure

Machang Type, Neolithic Age

Pottery

Mouth Diameter 19 cm/ Height 33.4 cm

This pot has a slightly flared mouth, a swelling belly with two ears. The front side of the pot is embossed with a portrait of human head on the upper part of the abdomen and a painted human body on the lower in relief. The reverse side is painted with frog patterns. Two flanks are adorned with a fishing-net design. It was excavated from Liupingtai in Liuwan Village, Qinghai Province.

Preserved in Liuwan Painted Pottery Museum, Qinghai Province

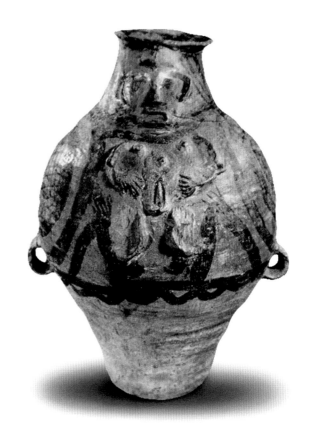

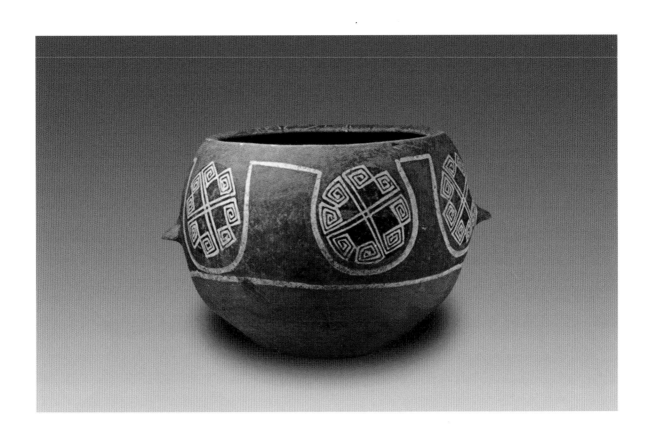

彩陶缶

新石器时代，大汶口文化

夹砂红陶质

口径 32 厘米，高 31 厘米

Painted Pottery "Fou" (Container)

Dawenkou Culture, Neolithic Age

Red Sandy Pottery

Mouth Diameter 32 cm/ Height 31 cm

施红色陶衣。敛口，折腹，平底，腹两侧装
鸭嘴形坠。腹上部用白彩绘"几"字纹与黑
地白色雷形几何纹。线条粗犷，题材新颖。
1974 年山东省泰安市大汶口出土。

山东省文物考古研究所藏

Covered with red coating, this container "Fou"
has a contracted mouth, an angular belly and a
flat bottom. Two duckbill-shaped handles are
attached to both sides of the belly. On the belly
are found some geometric patterns in the shape
of a Chinese character " 几 " in white and white
thunder patterns on a black background. Bold
lines and designs are drawn in a novel way. It
was excavated from Dawenkou Site of Taian
City, Shandong Province, in the year 1974.
Preserved in Institute of Cultural Relics and
Archaeology of Shandong Drovince

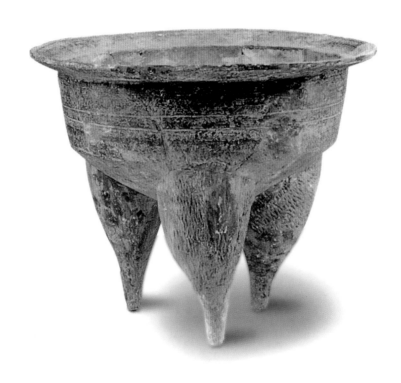

夹砂灰陶斝

新石器时代，河南龙山文化 (前 2600—前 2000)

夹砂灰陶质

口径 25 厘米，通高 20.5 厘米

Grey Sandy Pottery "Jia" (Drinking Vessel)

Longshan Culture of Henan Province (2600 B.C.–2000 B.C.), Neolithic Age

Grey Sandy Pottery

Mouth Diameter 25 cm/ Height 20.5 cm

此斝三足间形成的裆部分离较大，底部残存有烟炱痕迹。腹腔内有一层附着于器壁的白色垢迹，应系长期烧水形成的。河南省济源市原城遗址出土。

河南省文物考古研究院藏

On the bottom of this "Jia" (drinking vessel) is a wide-open space at the bottom among the three feet and traces of soot are visible. A layer of white incrustation adheres to the interior wall of the belly due to long-term exposure to boiling water. It was excavated from the Yuancheng Site in Jiyuan County, Henan Province.

Preserved in Henan Provincial Institute of Cultural Heritage and Archaeology

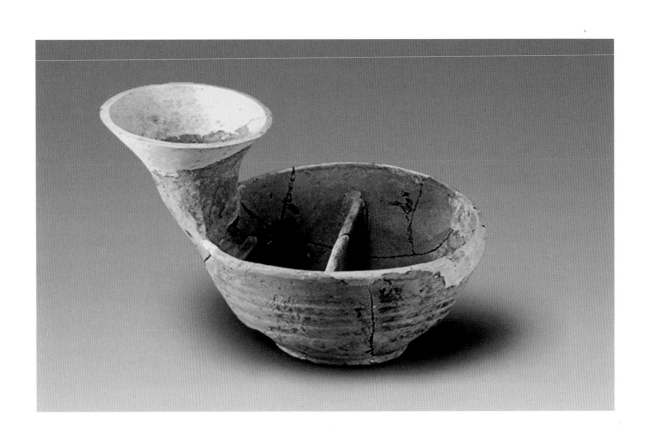

陶澄器

良渚文化

泥质灰陶质

通高 22 厘米

嘴：口径 15 厘米，高 10 厘米

器身：口径 23 厘米，高 12 厘米

圈足：底径 13 厘米

Pottery Clarifier

Liangzhu Culture

Grey Clay Pottery

Height 22 cm

Spout: Mouth Diameter 15 cm/ Height 10 cm

Body: Mouth Diameter 23 cm/ Height 12 cm

Ring Foot: Bottom Diameter 13 cm

器身中段有弦纹四道。这是一件实用器，器身中部有一竖向隔挡，低于口沿 2 厘米，澄清后的酒液可溢过隔挡流入另一半容器内。1982 年浙江省余杭吴家埠遗址出土。

浙江省文物考古研究所藏

Four bands of bow-string patterns are found in the middle of the abdomen. As a tool of practical use, the vessel has a vertical partition which is 2 cm lower than the rim. The clarified wine can flow over the partition into another half of this device. It was excavated from the Wujiabu Site in Yuhang City, Zhejiang Province.

Preserved in Institute of Cultural Relics and Archaeology of Zhejiang Province

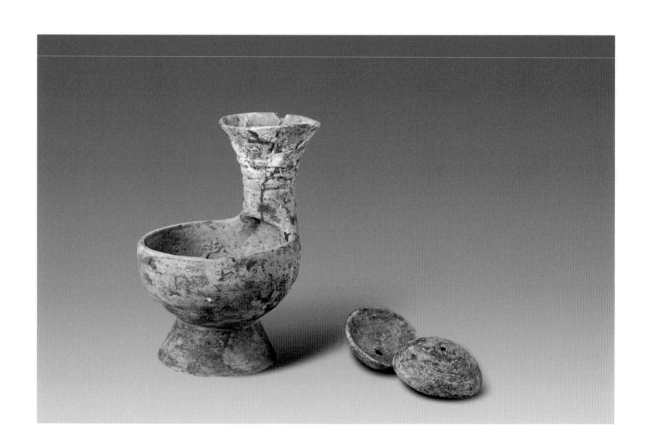

陶过滤器

良渚文化

泥质黑皮陶质

通高 16.8 厘米

盖：径 6.9 厘米，高 3 厘米

过滤钵：口径 6.2 厘米，高 2.5 厘米

嘴：口径 7 厘米，高 8 厘米

器身：口径 11.6 厘米，高 8.8 厘米

圈足：径 9.2 厘米

Pottery Filter

Liangzhu Culture

Black Clay Pottery

Height 16.8 cm

Lid: Diametre 6.9 cm/ Height 3 cm

Filter Bowl: Mouth Diameter 6.2 cm/ Height 2.5 cm

Spout: Mouth Diameter 7 cm/ Height 8 cm

Settling Device: Mouth Diameter 11.6 cm/ Height 8.8 cm

Ring Foot: Diametre 9.2 cm

全器由盖、过滤钵、澄器组成。盖为半球形，子母口。过滤钵为圜底，底中有一小孔，此为明器，小孔仅起滤孔的象征作用。澄器为口沿一侧安置一冲天嘴的钵形圈足器，冲天嘴敞口承接过滤钵，下端扁圆，与澄器相通。据实用器推测，此类造型奇特之陶器，似与制酒过程中澄清酒水的功能有关。1981 年浙江省余杭吴家埠遗址出土。

浙江省文物考古研究所藏

This filter is composed of a lid, a filter bowl and a clarifier. The lid is in the shape of a hemisphere, such that the closure may be snap-fit to a container neck. There is a small symbolic filter hole in the middle of the bottom since the vessel is a burial object. The clarifier, with an upward spout set on one side of the mouth rim, is a bowl-shaped device with a ring foot. The upward spout has a flared mouth to hold the filter bowl. The lower end of the spout is oblate in shape and connected to the clarifier. This type of pottery vessel with such a special design is presumed to serve as a filter to maintain the quality of water in making wine. It was excavated at the Wujiabu Site in Yuhang City, Zhejiang Province.

Preserved in Institute of Cultural Relics and Archaeology of Zhejiang Province

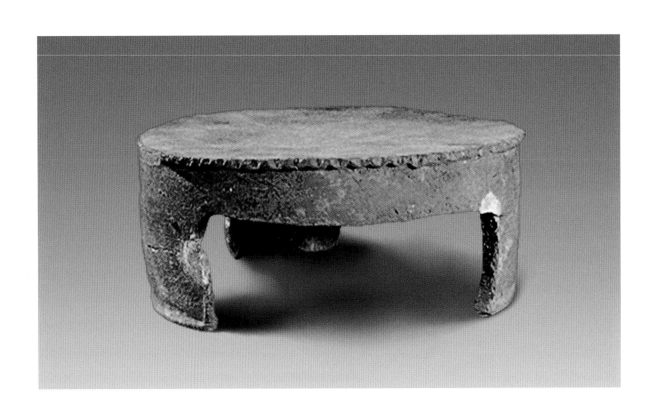

夹砂褐陶鏊

仰韶文化 (前 5000—前 3000)

夹砂褐陶质

直径 27 厘米，高 16 厘米

Brown Sandy Pottery Griddle

Yangshao Culture (5000 B.C.-3000 B.C.)

Brown Sandy Pottery

Diametre 27 cm/ Height 16 cm

一种制作饼类干食的器具。平面圆形，周边
有经过捏塑的泥条形成的附加堆纹。三条瓦
形足下部稍有内收，三足间形成的空间即置
薪烧柴的火门。用陶鏊烙饼的方法实际是对
旧石器时代晚期焙烧食品技法的继承和发展。
河南省荥阳市青台遗址出土。

郑州市文物考古研究院藏

The griddle is a flat-bottomed appliance for
making pies, the edge of which is decorated
with raised clay-stripes by hand kneading.
There are three tile-shaped feet turning slightly
inwards at the lower part. The spaces between
the feet serve as the vent of this griddle. Making
pancakes with pottery griddle is inherited from
baking techniques of the Upper Paleolithic. It
was excavated at the Qingtai Site of Xingyang
City, Henan Province.
Preserved in Institute of Cultural Relics and
Archaeology of Zhengzhou

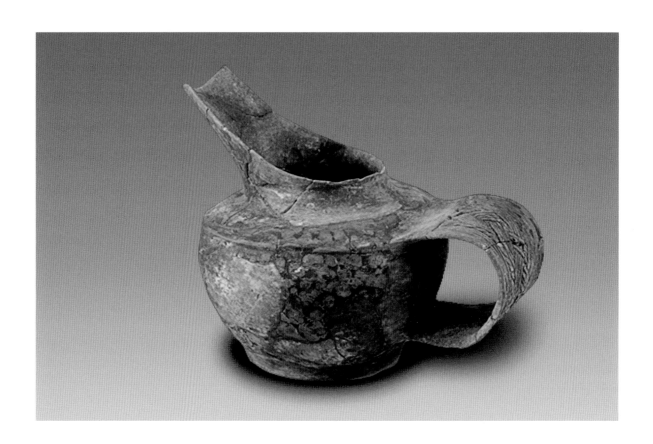

陶宽把壶

新石器时代

泥质灰黑陶质

口径 9.6 厘米，底径 11.4 厘米，高 20 厘米

Pottery Pot with Wide Handle

Neolithic Age

Greyish-black Clay Pottery

Mouth Diameter 9.6 cm/ Bottom Diameter 11.4 cm/ Height 20 cm

器身圆鼓，宽流高翘，矮圈足。器身饰浅细的篦划短线，纹样不明。宽鋬表面饰绞索状粗泥条贴塑纹。

海盐县博物馆藏

This pot has a globular body, a wide upward spout and a short ring foot. There are vague decorative patterns of short lines carved shallowly by grate bars on the abdomen. The wide handle surface is adorned with clay strips in noose shape.

Preserved in Haiyan Museum

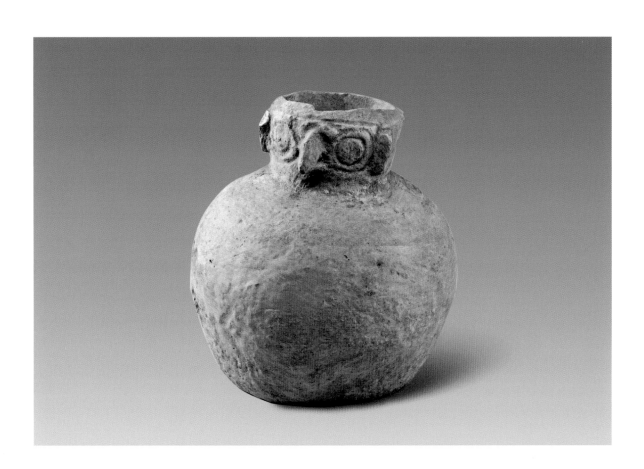

陶鹰头壶

崧泽文化

泥质灰陶质

口径 4 厘米，底径 7.6 厘米，高 11.6 厘米

Pot with Eagle-head Mouth

Songze Culture

Grey Clay Pottery

Mouth Diameter 4 cm/ Bottom Diameter 7.6 cm/ Height 11.6 cm

直口略残，平底。颈部堆塑刻画出一钩喙、
环眼、长耳的鹰隼头像。1996 年浙江省嘉兴
市南河浜遗址出土。

浙江省文物考古研究所藏

This pot has a slightly cracked straight mouth,
and a flat bottom. On the bottleneck is moulded
and carved an eagle head with a hooked beak,
round eyes and long ears in relief. It was
excavated from the Nanhebang Site of Jiaxing
City, Zhejiang Province, in the year 1996.
Preserved in Institute of Cultural Relics and
Archaeology of Zhejiang Province

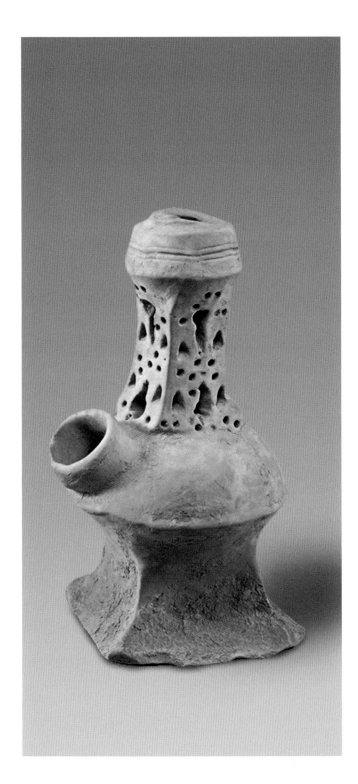

陶双口壶

崧泽文化

泥质红陶质

口径 3.6 ～ 4.6 厘米，底径 10.8 厘米，高
20 厘米

Pottery Pot with Double Mouths

Songze Culture

Red Clay Pottery

Mouth Diameter 3.6-4.6 cm/ Bottom Diameter

10.8 cm/ Height 20 cm

上口略残，呈蒜形，上刻凹弦纹。方颈，颈
上遍施圆形、三角形等镂孔。腹扁折，一侧
有一椭圆形直口。方形座，平底。该器头、颈、
腹部均中空，但互不相通。器形特殊，用途
不明。1996年浙江省嘉兴市南河浜遗址出土。

浙江省文物考古研究所藏

The pot's upper mouth, slightly cracked, is
garlic-shaped and decorated with concave bow-
string patterns. The square neck is covered
with circular and triangular fret-work. On one
side of the oblate and angular abdomen is set
another oval straight mouth. The pot sits on
a square pedestal with a flat bottom. There
is no connection between the cavities of the
head, neck and the belly. The pot is designed
with a special shape, but the function remains
unknown. It was excavated from the Nanhebang
Site of Jiaxing City, Zhejiang Province, in the
year 1996.

Preserved in Institute of Cultural Relics and
Archaeology of Zhejiang Province

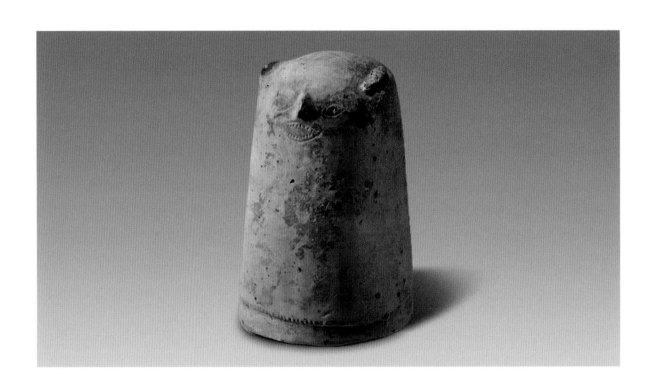

陶兽面壶

崧泽文化

泥质灰陶质

口径 2.4～4.4 厘米，底径 9 厘米，高 13.8 厘米

Pottery Pot with Animal Face Design

Songze Culture

Grey Clay Pottery

Mouth Diameter 2.4 - 4.4 cm/ Bottom Diameter 9 cm/ Height 13.8 cm

整器呈圆角方柱体。顶弧平，一侧堆塑刻划
一兽面：三角形鼻翼与扁条形兽耳用小泥块
堆塑，兽眼、嘴则用阴线刻划，还特意在眼
中点出眼珠，嘴里遍刻牙齿。另一侧则开一
椭圆形口。底宽平。1996 年浙江嘉兴市南河
浜遗址出土。

浙江省文物考古研究所藏

The whole vessel is shaped into a rounded
square cylinder. With a flat-top arc, this pot is
moulded and incised with an animal face on
one side. The animal face features a triangle
nose and flat bar-shaped ears moulded by clay
slates. By using the technique such as shade line
carving, the eyes and mouth are vividly carved,
including the eyeballs and teeth. On the other
side of the pot is set an oval-shaped mouth.
The bottom of the pot is broad and flat. It was
excavated from the Nanhebang Site of Jiaxing
City, Zhejiang Province, in the year 1996.
Preserved in Institute of Cultural Relics and
Archaeology of Zhejiang Province

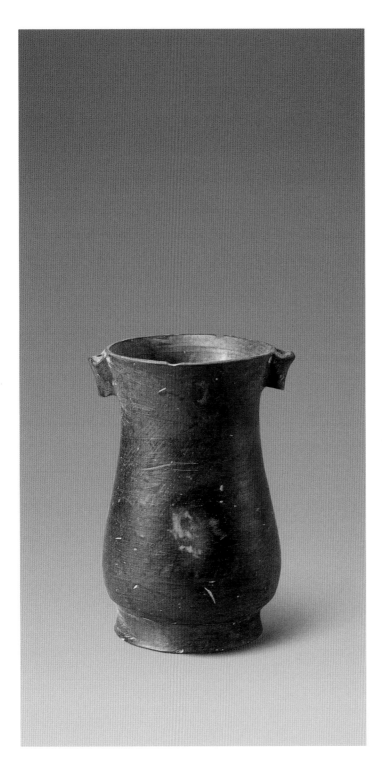

陶双鼻壶

良渚文化

泥质黑皮陶质

口径 6.2 厘米，底径 5.6 厘米，高
10.4 厘米

Pottery Pot with Double Noses

Liangzhu Culture

Black Clay Pottery

Mouth Diameter 6.2 cm/ Bottom

Diameter 5.6 cm/ Height 10.4 cm

黑皮铅色发亮。侈口，微鼓腹下坠，器形似杯。

口沿饰对称双鼻。器内壁可见多道轮制旋痕。

浙江省文物考古研究所藏

This pot is of black pottery coated with shiny leaden colour. It has a wide flared mouth and a slightly swelling and drooping abdomen. The pot is in the shape of a cup. There are two noses set symmetrically on either side of the mouth rim. The wheel-thrown curved scars can be seen in the interior wall.

Preserved in Institute of Cultural Relics and Archaeology of Zhejiang Province

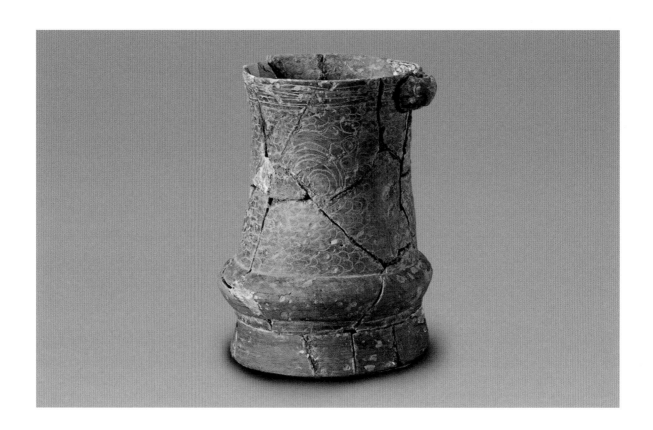

陶双鼻壶

良渚文化

泥质黑皮陶质

口径 6.8~7 厘米，底径 7.9 厘米，高 11.6 厘米

Pottery Pot with Double Noses

Liangzhu Culture

Black Clay Pottery

Mouth Diameter 6.8‑7 cm/ Bottom Diameter 7.9 cm/ Height 11.6 cm

扁腹，高圈足，为良渚文化中晚期的双鼻壶特征。壶颈部以阴线刻画蟠龙纹，龙体遍饰鳞纹。1995 年浙江省海宁市余墩庙出土。

浙江省文物考古研究所藏

This pot has an oblate abdomen and a high ring foot, which are the main features of the double-nosed pottery pot made during the middle and late period of the Liangzhu Culture. The pot neck is incised with a coiled dragon in shade lines. The dragon's body is covered with fish scale patterns. It was excavated from Yudun Temple of Haining City, Zhejiang Province, in the year 1995.

Preserved in Institute of Cultural Relics and Archaeology of Zhejiang Province

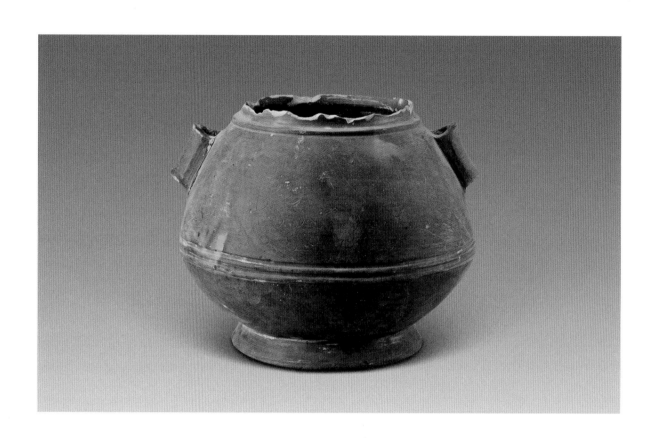

陶双鼻壶

良渚文化

泥质黑皮陶质

口径 6.8～7 厘米，底径 7.9 厘米，高 11.6 厘米

Pottery Pot with Double Noses

Liangzhu Culture

Black Clay Pottery

Mouth Diameter 6.8-7 cm/ Bottom Diameter 7.9 cm/ Height 11.6 cm

口稍残，颈部有一周凸棱。上腹部饰对称竖向贯耳，并以双耳为轴，两侧各浅刻一组由鸟首、羽翅和圆涡状卷曲蛇身构成的抽象图案。中腹另饰两周凹弦纹。

浙江省文物考古研究所藏

The pot mouth is slightly cracked, and a raised band can be seen around the neck.Two tube-shaped vertical handles are set at the symmetrical position of the upper abdomen, the sides of which are adorned with abstract depictions of bird heads, feathered wings, and whorl patterns of coiled snakes.
Preserved in Institute of Cultural Relics and Archaeology of Zhejiang Province

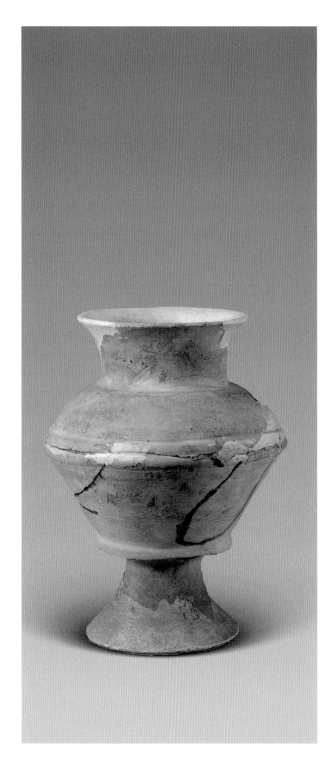

陶圈足壶

良渚文化

泥质灰陶质

壶：口径 9 厘米，底径 7.6 厘米，高 18 厘米

圈足：径 8.6 厘米，高 4.8 厘米

Pottery Pot with Ring Foot

Liangzhu Culture

Grey Clay Pottery

Pot: Mouth Diameter 9 cm/ Bottom Diameter 7.6 cm/

Height 18 cm

Ring Foot: Bottom Diameter 8.6 cm/ Height 4.8 cm

敞口，斜短颈，溜肩折腹，斜直腹内收成平底，底部加喇叭形圈足。制作规整，是良渚文化早期颇有特点的一种壶。1981年浙江省余杭吴家埠遗址出土。

浙江省文物考古研究所藏

This pot has an open mouth, a short slant neck, a sloping shoulder, an angular and oblique abdomen narrowing down to the flat bottom. The pot sits on a spreading trumpet-shaped base. It is made in a regular way with distinctive features of the early Liangzhu culture. It was excavated at Wujiabu Site of Yuhang City, Zhejiang Province, in the year 1981.

Preserved in Institute of Cultural Relics and Archaeology of Zhejiang Province

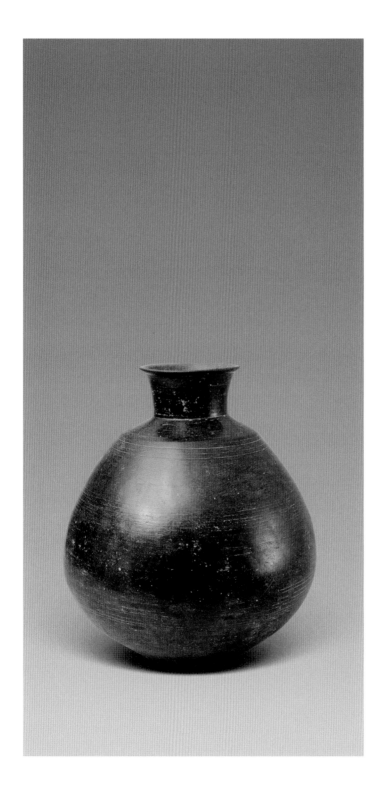

黑陶壶

新石器时代，龙山文化

泥质黑陶质

口径 11 厘米，高 30.5 厘米

Black Pottery Pot

Longshan Culture, Neolithic Age

Black Clay Pottery

Mouth Diameter 11 cm/ Height 30.5 cm

施黑陶衣，黑光发亮，轮制，侈口，口沿外卷，

颈高且直，折肩鼓腹，小平底。器型硕大，

盛水器。1977 年山东省寿光市火山埠出土。

寿光市博物馆藏

This pot is wheel-thrown and covered with
shiny black clay coating. It has a wide flared
mouth, an everted mouth rim, a high straight
neck, an angular shoulder, a swelling belly and
a small flat bottom. Large in size, the pot was
utilized as a water container. It was excavated
from the Site of Huoshanbu in Shouguang City,
Shandong Province, in the year 1977.

Preserved in Shouguang Museum

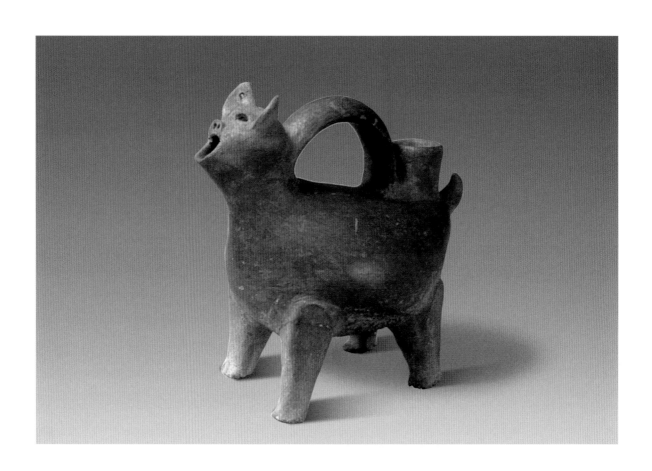

红陶兽形壶

新石器时代，大汶口文化

夹砂红陶质

长 22 厘米，宽 14 厘米，高 21.6 厘米

Red Pottery Pot in Animal Shape

Dawenkou Culture, Neolithic Age

Red Sandy Pottery

Length 22 cm/ Width 14 cm/ Height 21.6 cm

手工捏塑，压磨光滑，通体施红色陶衣。体形肥壮，圆面耸耳，拱鼻张口，四肢粗短有力，短尾上翘，似待食的小猪。尾部有筒形口可受水，嘴可注水，背安拱形鋬。造型生动，亦实用，惹人喜爱，是一件罕见珍品。1959 年山东省泰安市大汶口出土。

山东博物馆藏

This pot, with an entirely red pottery coating, was made through the technique of kneading and moulding, and then was pressed and polished into smooth-surfaced pottery. The pot is shaped like a piglet waiting to be fed. The piglet has a stout and strong body, a round face with two erect ears, a typical hog nose, an open mouth, four stubby limbs and a short tail curling upward. There is a cylindrical wide mouth on the rear part of the piglet body for filling in water, and an arc-shaped handle is set on the piglet back. The design of the pot is vivid, endearing and functional, making it a rare treasure. It was excavated from Dawenkou Site of Taian City, Shandong Province, in the year 1959.

Preserved in Shandong Museum

彩陶罐

新石器时代，马家窑文化 (前 3300—前 2050)

陶质

口径 13 厘米，高 28.5 厘米

Painted Pottery Pot

Majiayao Culture (3300 B.C.-2050 B.C.), Neolithic Age

Pottery

Mouth Diameter 13 cm/ Height 28.5 cm

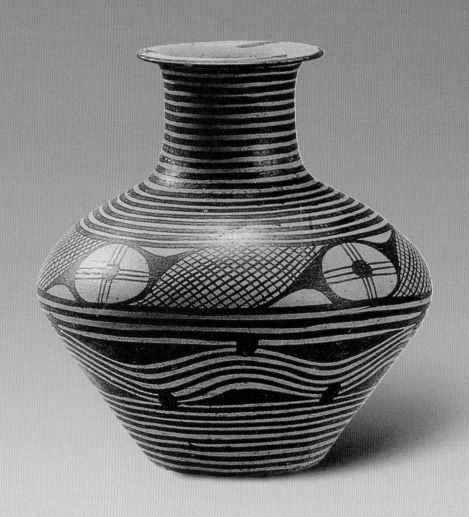

新石器时代的重要盛贮器。敞口细颈，既便于盛贮物品的向内灌注，又防止了向外的溅溢，浑圆的深腹又增加了容量及重心的稳固，造型设计准确地体现了其用途。青海省民和县出土。

青海省文物考古研究所藏

This pottery pot was a kind of container that was widely used in the Neolithic Age. It is designed with an open mouth and a slender bottleneck, with which water will be filled in without spill. The deep circular belly can increase the capacity and the stability of the pot. The design and the shape of this pot indicate clearly the function of it. It was excavated from Minhe County, Qinghai Province.

Preserved in Institute of Cultural Relics and Archaeology of Qinghai Province

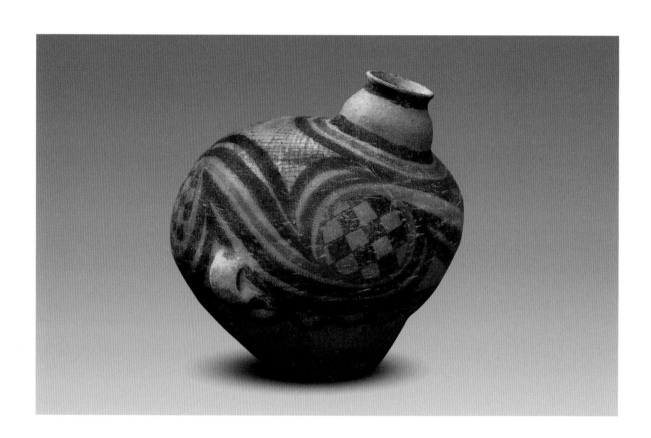

彩陶壶

新石器时代，马家窑文化半山类型

陶质

口径 6 厘米，底径 10 厘米，通高 26.5 厘米

Painted Pottery Pot

Majiayao Culture, Banshan Type, Neolithic Age

Pottery

Mouth Diameter 6 cm/ Bottom Diameter 10 cm/ Height 26.5 cm

平底，鼓腹，双耳，后腹部有把。口外侧口
沿向外撇。腹部饰有黑红两彩的弧线三角条
带，条带间隔饰圆形网格图案。生活与卫生
器物。

郭鹏云供稿

This painted pottery pot has a flat bottom, a
globular body with two ears, a handle attached
to the rear of the belly, and a flaring mouth
rim. The belly is decorated with black and red
curved lines with triangles. The space within
the lines is filled up with net patterns. It was
utilized as a daily living and hygiene utensil.
Submitted by Guo Pengyun

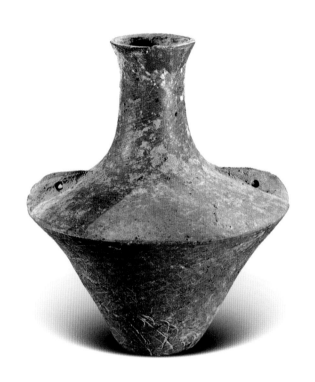

红陶折肩壶

新石器时代早期，裴李岗文化（前 5500—前 4900)

红陶质

口径 4.6 厘米，高 17.6 厘米

河南省长葛市石固遗址出土。

河南省文物考古研究院藏

Red Pottery Pot with Angular Shoulder

Peiligang Culture in the early Neolithic Age (5500 B.C. – 4900 B.C.)

Red Pottery

Mouth Diameter 4.6 cm/ Height 17.6 cm

The pot was excavated at the Shigu Site of Changge City, Henan Province.

Preserved in Henan Provincial Institute of Cultural Heritage and Archaeology

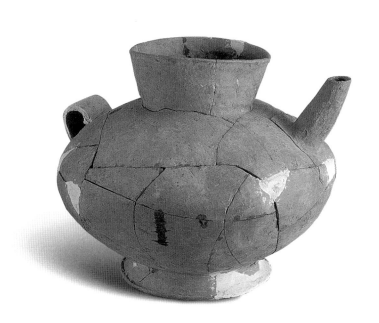

硬陶盉

马桥文化

陶质

口径 10 厘米，底径 11.6 厘米，高 17.2 厘米

遂昌县文物管理委员会藏

Hard Pottery "He" (Drinking Vessel)

Maqiao Culture

Pottery

Mouth Diameter 10 cm/ Bottom Diameter 11.6 cm/ Height 17.2 cm

Preserved in Department of Cultural Relics Coneservation of Suichang County

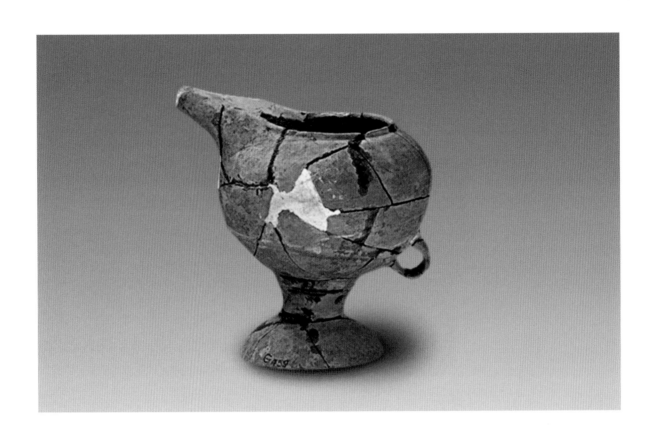

豆形陶盉

新石器时代

泥质灰胎

口径 9.5 厘米，腹径 14.3 厘米，通高 18.8 厘米

Bean-shaped Pottery "He" (Drinking Vessel)

Neolithic Age

Clay Pottery with Grey Body

Mouth Diameter 9.5 cm/ Belly Diameter 14.3 cm/ Height 18.8 cm

卷口，球腹，矮把，喇叭形底座。江苏省
南京市高淳区固城镇朝墩头遗址出土。

高淳区文物保管所藏

The vessel has a scroll-shaped mouth, a
ball-shaped belly, a handle attached to the
lower part of the belly and a trumpet-shaped
pedestal. Its grey body is made of clay. It was
unearthed from Chaoduntou Site, Gucheng
Town, Gaochun District, Nanjing City,
Jiangsu Province.

Preserved in Cultural Relics Preservation of
Gaochun District

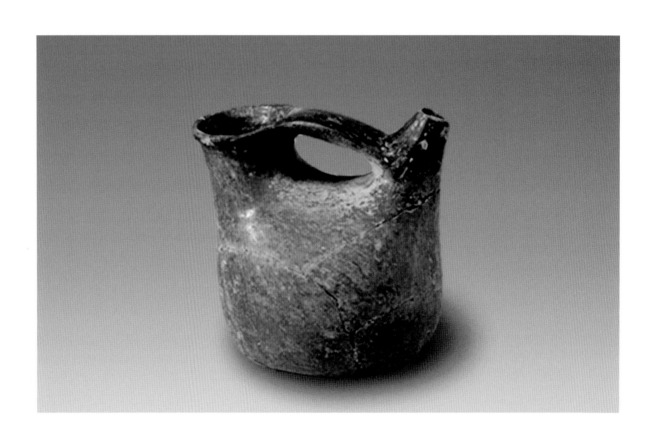

垂囊盉

河姆渡文化

陶质

底径 12.6 厘米，通高 17.9 厘米

Pendulous-bag-shaped "He" (Drinking Vessel)

Hemudu Culture

Pottery

Bottom Diameter 12.6 cm/ Height 17.9 cm

酒器。泥质红衣陶，前嘴后注，河姆渡文化
特色器型。1996 年浙江省余姚市鲻山遗址
出土。

浙江省文物考古研究所藏

The vessel served as a wine container. With a
red clay body, a front spout and a rear filling
opening, it was a distinctive representative of
the Hemudu Culture. It was unearthed from
Zishan Site, Yuyao City, Zhejiang Province, in
the year 1996.

Preserved in Institute of Cultural Relics and
Archaeology of Zhejiang Province

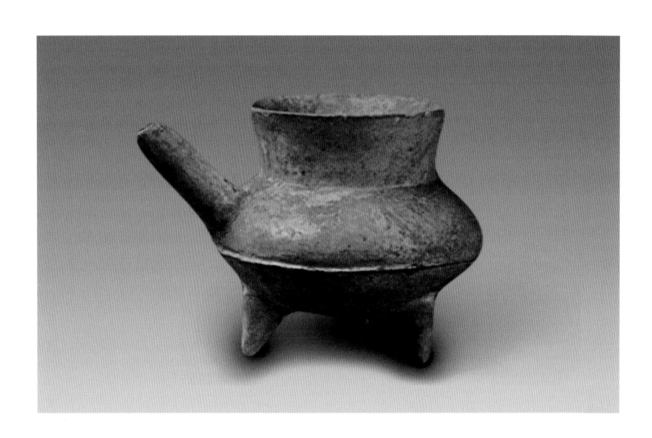

白陶三足盉

新石器时代，大汶口文化

陶质

口径 13 厘米，高 15.4 厘米

White Pottery Tripod "He" (Drinking Vessel)

Dawenkou Culture, Neolithic Age

Pottery

Mouth Diameter 13 cm/ Height 15.4 cm

用高岭土做原料，胎质细腻，手工成型，器壁较薄，施白陶衣光润洁白。侈口，粗颈，扁圆腹，小平底，安凿形实足，肩一侧装上翘的管状流。腹部饰有凸棱。盉可盛水或酒。造型端庄，工艺精致，属新石器时代白陶中的精品，为商周白陶工艺的高度发展奠定了技术基础。1959 年山东省泰安市大汶口出土。

山东博物馆藏

The vessel body is made of Kaolin clay, exquisite in texture. It is manually shaped and has a thin wall with a white coating, which looks smooth and pure. The vessel has a flared mouth, a broad neck, an oval-shaped belly and a small flat bottom. To the bottom are attached scalpriform feet and on the shoulder is an upward tubular spout. A convex ridge can be seen on its belly. "He" is used as water or wine containers. With an elegant shape and exquisite craftsmanship, it is a masterpiece of white pottery of the Neolithic Age and had laid the foundation for the future development of white pottery craftsmanship in the Shang and the Zhou Dynasty. The vessel was unearthed from Dawenkou Site, Tai'an City, Shandong Province, in the year 1959.

Preserved in Shandong Museum

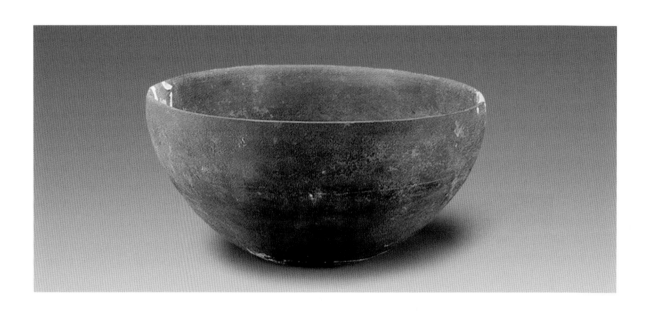

红陶钵

新石器时代，仰韶文化

陶质

口径 30.5 厘米，高 16.5 厘米，重 750 克

底残损，是当时的生活器物。陕西省西安市沪河遗址出土。

陕西医史博物馆藏

Red Pottery Bowl

Yangshao Culture, Neolithic Age

Pottery

Mouth Diameter 30.5 cm/ Height 16.5 cm/ Weight 750 g

The vessel served as a household utensil at that time and its bottom was damaged. It was unearthed from the Chanhe River ruins, Xi'an City, Shaanxi Province.

Preserved in Shaanxi Museum of Medical History

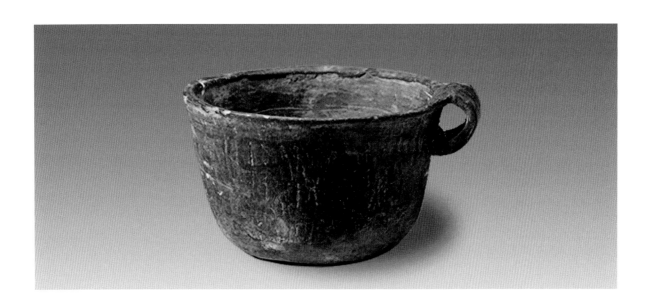

单把钵

河姆渡文化

陶质

口径 16.2 厘米，底径 8.8 厘米，高 9.4 厘米

1996 年浙江省余姚市鲻山遗址出土。

浙江省文物考古研究所藏

Single-handled Bowl

Hemudu Culture

Pottery

Mouth Diameter 16.2 cm/ Bottom Diameter 8.8 cm/ Height 9.4 cm

This bowl was unearthed from Zishan Site, Yuyao City, Zhejiang Province, in the year 1996.

Preserved in Institute of Cultural Relics and Archaeology of Zhejiang Province

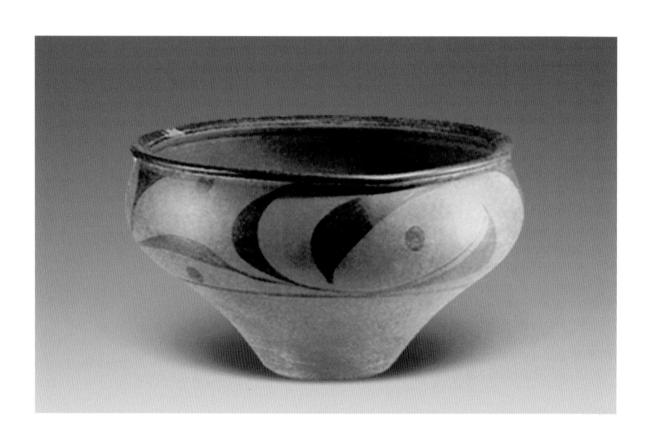

勾叶纹彩陶钵

仰韶文化（前 5000—前 3000)

陶质

口径 35.5 厘米，底径 13.5 厘米，高 24 厘米

Painted Pottery Bowl with Leaf Designs

Yangshao Culture (5000 B.C. – 3000 B.C.)

Pottery

Mouth Diameter 35.5 cm/ Bottom Diameter 13.5 cm/ Height 24 cm

此钵造型极具实用意义，构图简洁，色调和谐，笔触洗练，是庙底沟类型仰韶文化彩陶中的上佳之作。盛水器皿。1979年山西省方山遗址出土。

山西省考古研究所藏

The shape of this bowl suggests great functional value, and it served as a water container. With simple motifs, harmonious colours and neat lines and styles, it is a masterpiece of the painted pottery of Miaodigou Type, Yangshao Culture. The vessel was unearthed from Fangshan ruins, Shanxi Province, in the year 1979.

Preserved in Shanxi Provincial Institute of Archaeology

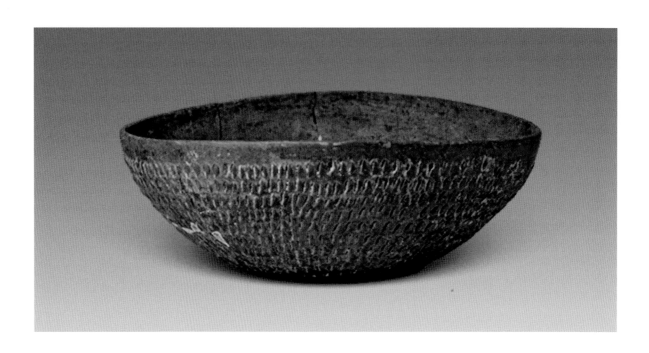

指甲纹红陶钵

新石器时代，北辛文化

泥质红陶质

口径 20.1 厘米，高 7.1 厘米

Red Pottery Bowl with Fingernail Patterns

Beixin Culture, Neolithic Age

Red Clay Pottery

Mouth Diameter 20.1 cm/ Height 7.1 cm

手工成型。大口微敛，腹部内收，水平底。周身饰指甲纹，排列有序。钵是当时居民常用的饮食器皿。1979 年山东省滕州市北辛村出土。

滕州博物馆藏

This bowl is made of clay with a red coating. It is manually shaped and has a large and slightly contracted mouth, an inward-contracted belly and a flat bottom. Its exterior wall is decorated orderly with fingernail patterns. The bowl was used as a food utensil at that time and it was unearthed from Beixin Village, Tengzhou City, Shandong Province, in the year 1979.

Preserved in Tengzhou Museum

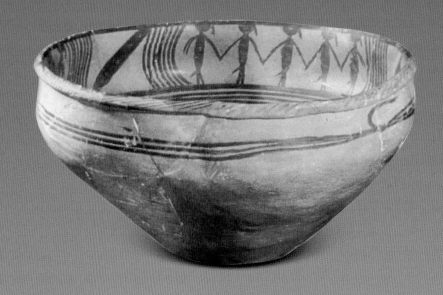

舞蹈纹彩陶盆

新石器时代，马家窑文化

陶质

口径 28.5 厘米，高 12.7 厘米

Painted Pottery Basin with Dancing Figures

Majiayao Culture, Neolithic Age

Pottery

Mouth Diameter 28.5 cm/ Height 12.7 cm

盆内壁有 5 人一组、手拉手的舞蹈纹饰，生
动地表现了先民们以舞蹈抒发感情、锻炼身
体的情景。1973 年青海大通县孙家寨出土。

青海省博物馆藏

On the interior wall of the basin are painted
patterns of groups of five figures dancing hand
in hand. It vividly depicts how the residents
expressed their feelings and built up their bodies
through dancing at that time. The basin was
unearthed from Sunjiazhai of Datong County,
Qinghai Province, in the year 1973.

Preserved in Qinghai Province Museum

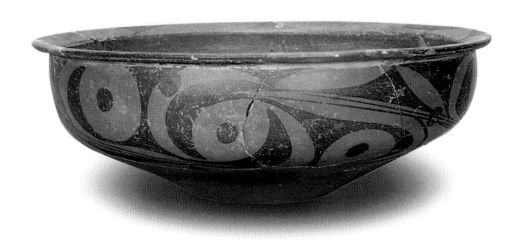

彩陶曲腹盆

新石器时代，仰韶文化庙底沟类型（前 4000—前 3000)

陶质

口径 40 厘米，高 13.8 厘米

Painted Pottery Basin with Angular Belly

Miaodigou Type, Yangshao Culture, Neolithic Age (4000 B.C. – 3000 B.C.)

Pottery

Mouth Diameter 40 cm/ Height 13.8 cm

敞口而深曲腹。盆的外表遍施红彩为底色即
"陶衣"，其上用黑彩绘出二方连续几何纹样，
造型和构图为庙底沟类型的典型风格。色泽、
线条与布局的匠心，代表了这一时期彩陶艺
术的最高成就。古代食具。陕西华县泉护遗
址出土。

北京大学赛克勒考古与艺术博物馆藏

The basin has a flared mouth and a deep angular
belly. Its exterior wall is covered with red-
grounding known as the "pottery coating".
Above the red coating are painted consecutive
geometric patterns in black. The shape of the
basin and the design of the patterns are typical
of the Miaodigou Culture. With ingenious
colours, lines and designs, the basin represents
the highest achievement in painted pottery
craftsmanship at that time. It served as a food
container and was unearthed from Quanhu Site,
Huaxian County, Shaanxi Province.
Preserved in Arthur M. Sackler Museum of Art
and Archaeology at Peking University

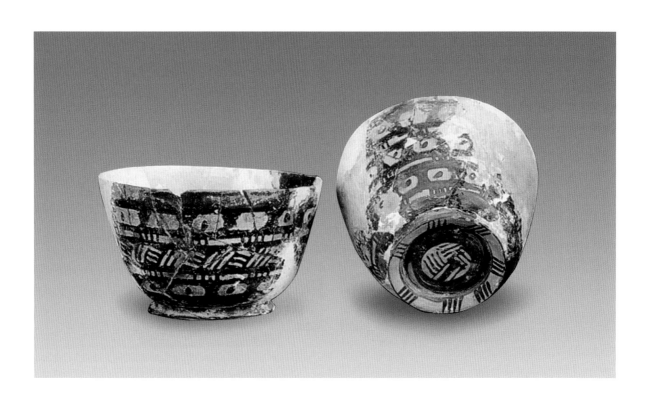

蛋壳形彩陶碗 (一对)

大溪文化

陶质

口径 11 厘米，底径 6.4~7 厘米，通高 8.5~8.7
厘米

荆州博物馆藏

**A Pair of Painted Eggshell-shaped
Pottery Bowls**

Daxi Culture

Pottery

Mouth Diameter 11 cm/ Bottom Diameter 6.4‑7 cm/

Height 8.5‑8.7 cm

Preserved in Jingzhou Museum

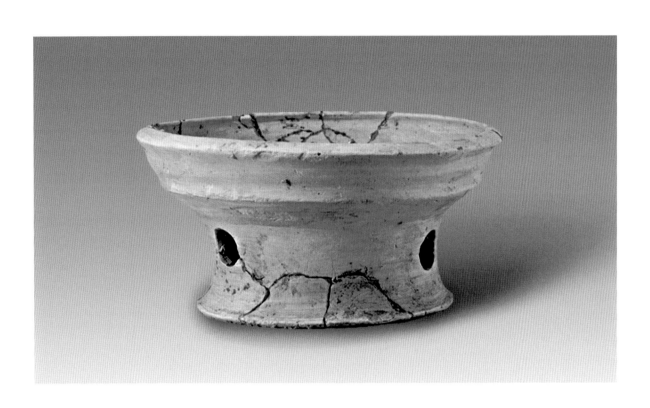

陶圈足盘

良渚文化

泥质黄胎灰黑陶质

口径 17 厘米，底径 13.6 厘米，高 9.2 厘米

盘腹外壁起二道凹弧。圈足上饰三个镂孔。

浙江省文物考古研究所藏

Pottery Ring-foot Plate

Liangzhu Culture

Clay Pottery

Mouth Diameter 17 cm/ Bottom Diameter 13.6 cm/ Height 9.2 cm

The plate has a yellow clayish body and a greyish-black coating. On its exterior wall are two circles of concave rings and on its ring foot are engraved three openings.

Preserved in Institute of Cultural Relics and Archaeology of Zhejiang Province

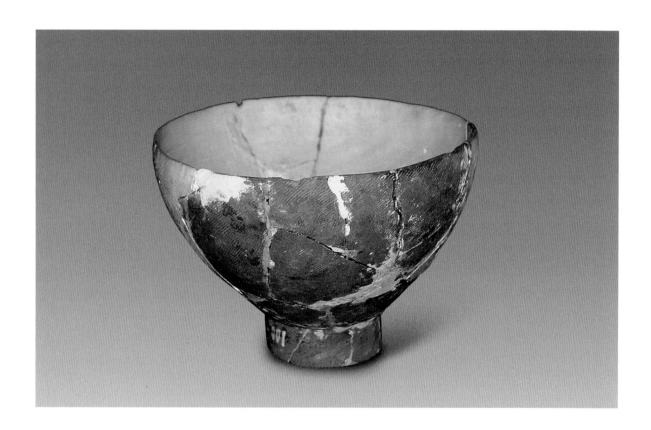

陶碗

新石器时代

陶质

口径 17.5 厘米，底径 6.5 厘米，通高 12.5 厘米，重 400 克

Pottery Bowl

Neolithic Age

Pottery

Mouth Diameter 17.5 cm/ Bottom Diameter 6.5 cm/ Height 12.5 cm/ Weight 400 g

敞口，斜腹，高圈足，周身细绳纹。食器，
有修补。陕西省西安市征集。

陕西医史博物馆藏

The bowl has a flared mouth, a sloping belly
and a high ring foot. It is decorated with thin
cord patterns. It was used as a food utensil and
has been restored. The bowl was collected from
Xi'an City, Shaanxi Province.

Preserved in Shaanxi Museum of Medical History

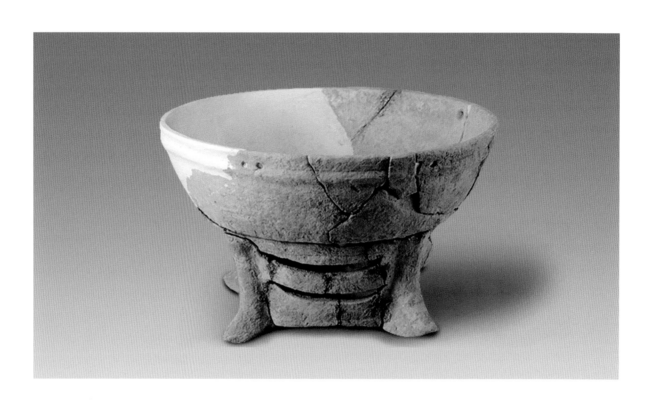

陶圈足盘

良渚文化

陶质

口径 17.5 厘米，高 10.3 厘米

Pottery Plate with Ring Foot

Liangzhu Culture

Pottery

Mouth Diameter 17.5 cm/ Height 10.3 cm

泥质黑皮陶，圆盘，方形圈足。圈足每边各
镂两个狭长的月牙形孔，四角则各贴塑人脚
形支腿。

浙江省文物考古研究所藏

The plate has a clayish body and a black
coating. It consists of a round plate and a
rectangular ring foot. Two long and narrow
crescent-shaped openings are engraved on each
side of the ring foot and human-foot-shaped
legs are sculpted and pasted on its four corners.
Preserved in Institute of Cultural Relics and
Archaeology of Zhejiang Province

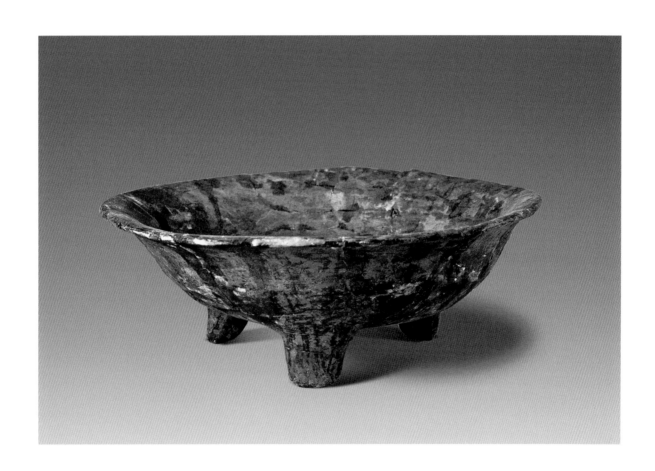

黑陶三足盘

马桥文化

泥质灰胎黑皮陶质

口径 22 厘米，高 7.6 厘米

Black Pottery Tripod Plate

Maqiao Culture

Clay Pottery

Mouth Diameter 22 cm/ Height 7.6 cm

出土时乌黑发亮，盘沿和三足正面中部施朱
彩。1997 年浙江省遂昌好川墓地出土。

遂昌县文物管理委员会藏

The plate has a grey clayish body and a
black coating. It was in lustrous black when
unearthed. The plate's rim and the forefront
centres of its three feet are painted vermilion.
It was unearthed from the tombs of Haochuan
Village, Suichang County, Zhejiang Province,
in 1997.
Preserved in Department of Cultural Relics
Coneservation of Suichang County

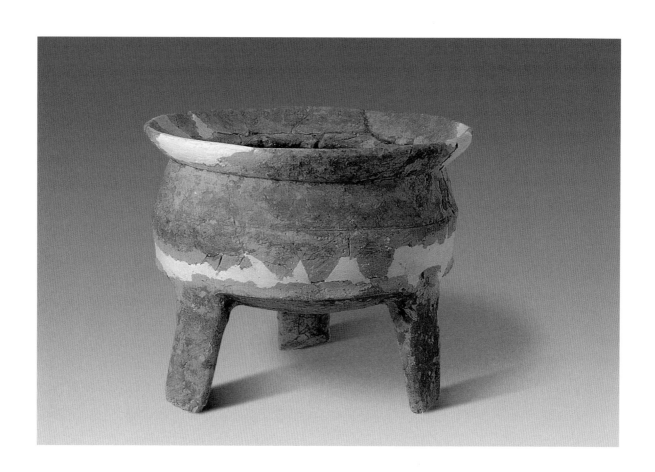

泥质灰陶三足盘

马桥文化

灰陶质

口径 15.8 厘米，高 12.5 厘米

Grey Clay Pottery Tripod Plate

Maqiao Culture

Grey Pottery

Mouth Diameter 15.8 cm/ Height 12.5 cm

1997 年浙江省遂昌好川墓地出土。

遂昌县文物管理委员会藏

The plate was unearthed from the tombs of Haochuan

Village, Suichang County, Zhejiang Province, in the

year 1997.

Preserved in Department of Cultural Relics

Coneservation of Suichang County

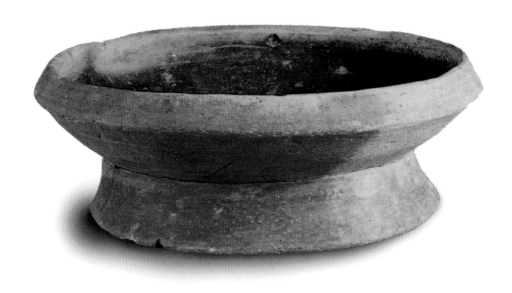

红陶圈足盘

新石器时代晚期，大溪文化 (前 4400 —前 3000)

红陶质

口径 18.8 厘米，高 6.7 厘米

Red Pottery Ring-foot Plate

Daxi Culture (4400 B.C. – 3000 B.C.), Late Neolithic Age

Red Pottery

Mouth Diameter 18.8 cm/ Height 6.7 cm

造型奇特，硬朗稳健。上古时用来盛放食品的器皿。湖北省宜都市红花套遗址出土。

北京大学赛克勒考古与艺术博物馆藏

The plate is unique in shape, and looks solid and strong. It was used as a food container in ancient times. It was unearthed from Honghuatao Site, Yidu City, Hubei Province. Preserved in Arthur M. Sackler Museum of Art and Archaeology at Peking University

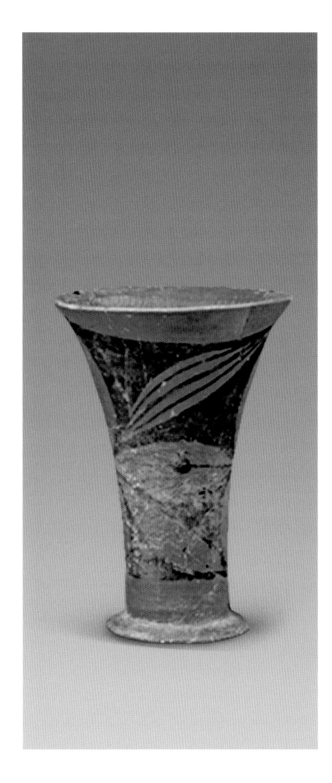

花瓣纹彩陶觚

新石器时代，大汶口文化

泥质红陶质

口径 12.2 厘米，高 16.5 厘米

Painted Pottery "Gu" (Vessel) with Petal Patterns

Dawenkou Culture, Neolithic Age

Red Clay Pottery

Mouth Diameter 12.2 cm/ Height 16.5 cm

通体施红色陶衣。喇叭形口，深腹，平底。
腹部绘有黑色树叶花瓣纹。红底黑彩，热烈
庄重。山东省兖州市王因村出土。

济宁博物馆藏

The vessel is made of clay and is covered with
red coating. It has a trumpet mouth, a deep belly
and a flat bottom. On its belly are painted black
leaf patterns and petal patterns, which look
enthusiastic and solemn against the red ground.
The vessel was unearthed from Wangyin
Village, Yanzhou City, Shandong Province.
Preserved in Jining Museum

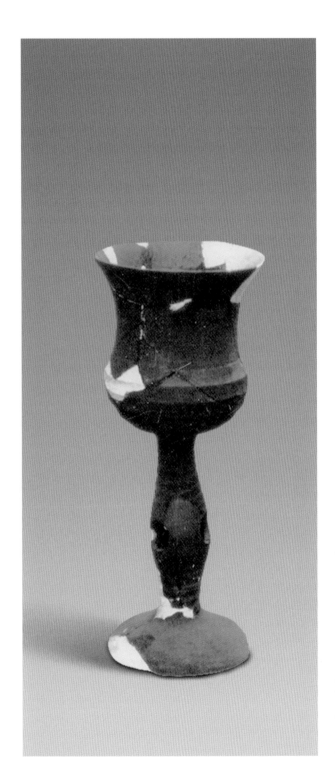

黑陶高柄杯

新石器时代

黑陶质

Black Pottery Goblet

Neolithic Age

Black Pottery

极似现代使用的高脚杯，大汶口文化酒具之
一。1971 年于山东邹县野店遗址出土。

山东博物馆藏

This vessel is very much similar to a modern
goblet and belongs to a type of wine container
in the Dawenkou Culture. It was unearthed from
Yedian Site, Zou County, Shandong Province,
in the year 1971.

Preserved in Shandong Museum

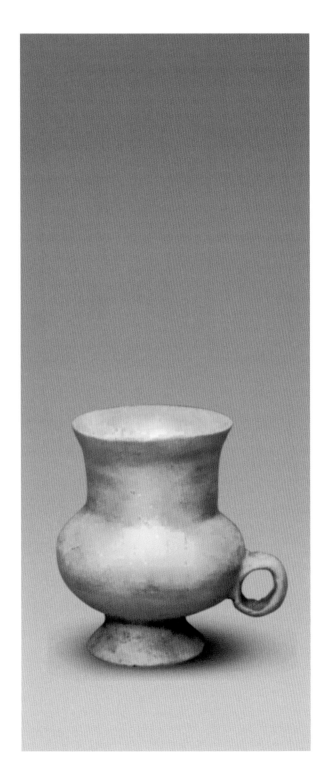

白陶单耳杯

新石器时代

陶质

White Pottery Cup with Single Ear

Neolithic Age

Pottery

该藏以高岭土做原料，胎质细腻，色泽皎白，是大汶口文化时期最典型的珍稀物品之一。多属酒具一类。自古以来，酒与医药有密切关系。1959年于山东省泰安市大汶口遗址出土。

山东博物馆藏

The cup is one of the rare items most typical of Dawenkou Culture Period. With kaoline as its raw material, the body of the cup is fine and smooth, casting a white lustre. It served as a wine container. Wine has been closely related to traditional Chinese medicines since ancient times. It was unearthed from the Dawenkou Site in Tai'an, Shandong Province, in the year 1959.

Preserved in Shandong Museum

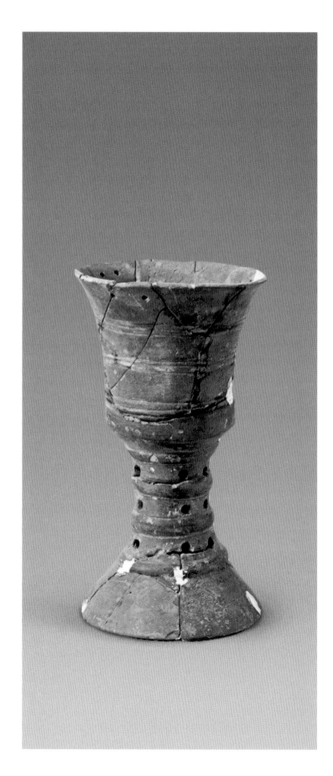

陶高足杯

崧泽文化

泥质黑皮陶质

口径 10.8 厘米，底径 10.8 厘米，高 18.2 厘米

Pottery Goblet

Songze Culture

Black Clay Pottery

Mouth Diameter 10.8 cm/ Bottom Diameter 10.8 cm/

Height 18.2 cm

深腹，高圈足。

浙江省文物考古研究所藏

The cup has a deep belly and a high ring foot.
Preserved in Institute of Cultural Relics and
Archaeology of Zhejiang Province

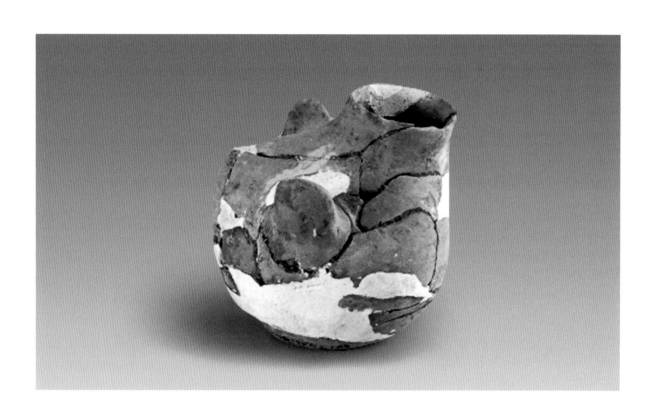

陶鸭形杯

崧泽文化晚期良渚文化早期

泥质灰陶质

口径 4 厘米，底径 5.3 厘米

Duck-shaped Pottery Cup

Late Songze Culture / Early Liangzhu Culture

Grey Clay Pottery

Mouth Diameter 4 cm/ Bottom Diameter 5.3 cm

似小鸭形，饰双翅，平底。1996 年浙江省海盐龙潭港遗址出土。

海盐县博物馆藏

The cup is a piece of grey clay pottery with a flat bottom. It looks like a duckling decorated with two wings. It was unearthed from the Longtan Port Site, Haiyan County, Zhejiang Province, in the year 1996.

Preserved in Haiyan Museum

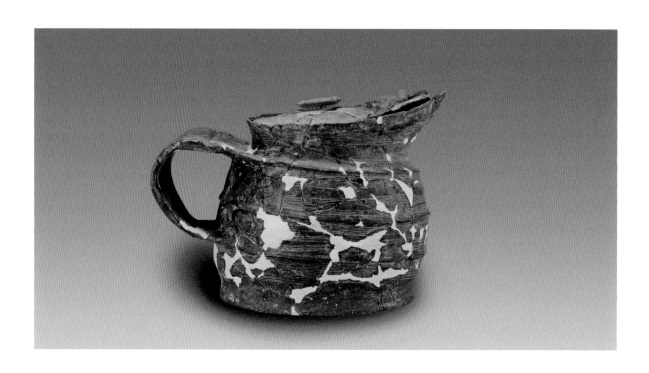

陶宽把杯

良渚文化

夹细砂黑皮陶质

口径 14 厘米，底径 14.6 厘米，高 15.2 厘米

Pottery Cup with Wide Handle

Liangzhu Culture

Black Sandy Pottery

Mouth Diameter 14 cm/ Bottom Diameter 14.6 cm/ Height 15.2 cm

器身粗大，带流、带盖，矮圈足。宽把表面由数十根细泥条贴塑。流下侧、器身及宽把上侧分别饰不同的怪异动物纹样刻划纹，为以往良渚文化所罕见。

海盐县博物馆藏

The cup, a piece of black pottery mixed with fine sand, has a bulky body, a spout, a lid and a short ring foot. On the surface of the wide handle are pasted about dozens of thin strips made of clay. Designs of various weird animals are carved below the spout, on the belly and the upper side of the wide handle, which is very rare in Liangzhu Culture.

Preserved in Haiyan Museum

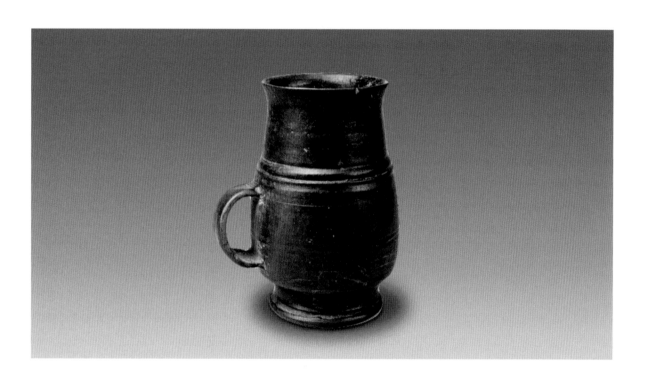

黑陶单把杯

新石器时代，龙山文化

泥质黑陶质

口径 5.9 厘米，足径 5.2 厘米，高 10.5 厘米

Black Pottery Cup with Single Handle

Longshan Culture, Neolithic Age

Black Clay Pottery

Mouth Diameter 5.9 cm/ Foot Diametre 5.2 cm/ Height 10.5 cm

轮制成型，施黑陶衣。侈口，高颈，深腹微鼓，
平底接矮圈足，附带式柄。造型朴实、实用。
1977 年山东省临沂市大范庄出土。

临沂市博物馆藏

The cup, covered with black pottery coating,
was made on a rotating wheel. It has a flared
mouth, a high neck, a deep and slightly bulging
belly, a flat bottom, sitting on a short ring foot.
A belt-shaped handle is attached to the body of
the cup. The cup is simple in design and easy to
use. It was unearthed from Dafanzhuang Village
in Linyi, Shandong Province, in the year 1977.
Preserved in Linyi Museum

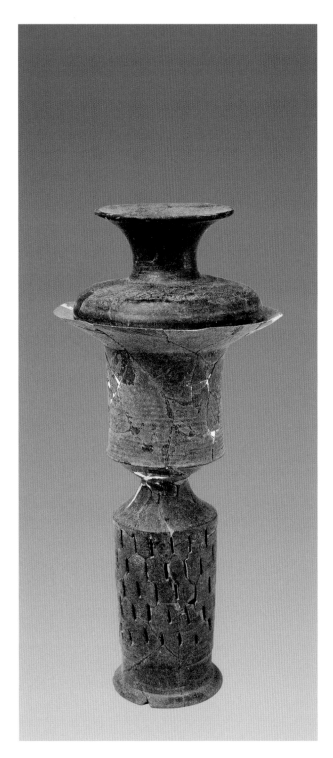

蛋壳黑陶盖杯

新石器时代，龙山文化

泥质黑陶质

口径 9 厘米，足径 4.7 厘米，通高 19.5 厘米

Eggshell-thin Black Pottery Cup with Cover

Longshan Culture, Neolithic Age

Black Clay Pottery

Mouth Diameter 9 cm/ Foot Diametre 4.7 cm/

Height 19.5 cm

轮制成型，壁薄体轻。宽口沿，深腹，圆底，下附高柄，柄作圆筒状，矮圈足。器上有通心覆豆式盖。柄部饰竖长条镂孔。酒杯有盖，可保持杯内清洁。1980 年山东省临沂市罗庄镇湖西崖村出土。

临沂市博物馆藏

The cup, made on a rotating wheel, has a thin wall and a light body. It distinguishes itself with a wide rim, a deep belly, a round bottom, a high cylinder-shaped handle and a short ring foot. Its cover looks like an upside-down stemmed cup, hollow inside. Its handle is decorated with vertical long holes. The cover on its top works well to keep the cup clean. It was unearthed from Huxiya Village in Luozhuang Town, Linyi City, Shandong Province in the year 1980.

Preserved in Linyi Museum

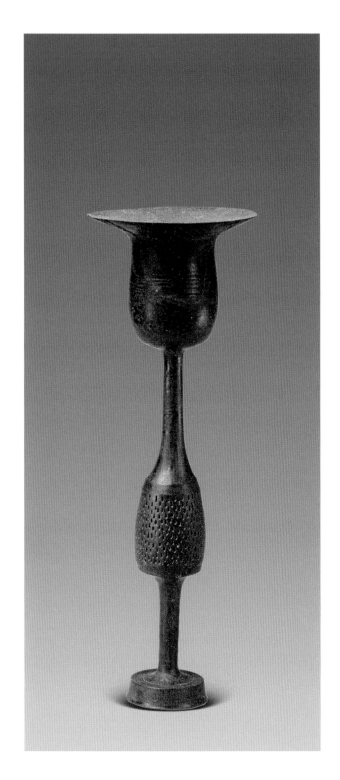

蛋壳黑陶高柄杯

新石器时代，龙山文化

泥质黑陶质

口径 9.4 厘米，足径 4.7 厘米，高 26.5 厘米，

重 93 克

Eggshell-thin Black Pottery Cup with High Stem

Longshan Culture, Neolithic Age

Black Clay Pottery

Mouth Diameter 9.4 cm/ Foot Diametre 4.7 cm/

Height 26.5 cm/ Weight 93 g

轮制成型。宽口沿，深腹，圈底，细高柄。柄作管状，中部外鼓，下部作台形圈足。柄饰楔形镂孔。壁薄如蛋壳，乌黑发亮，装饰素雅，属高级饮酒器。

山东省文物考古研究所藏

This cup is a piece of argillaceous black pottery. It is wheel-thrown, and featured with a wide edge, a deep belly, a round bottom and a tall thin stem. The stem is in the shape of a tube but bulging in the middle,and its lower part is a stand-shaped ring foot. The handle is decorated with wedged hollowed-out holes. The wall of the cup is as thin as the eggshell. It is a high-grade drinking vessel in lustrous black, with simple but elegant design.

Preserved in Institute of Cultural Relics and Archaeology of Shandong Drovince

新石器时代，龙山文化

泥质黑陶质

口径 14.2 厘米，足径 6.1 厘米，通高 12.4 厘米

Eggshell-thin Black Pottery Retainer Cup

Longshan Culture, Neolithic Age

Black Clay Pottery

Mouth Diameter 14.2 cm/ Foot Diametre 6.1 cm/ Height 12.4 cm

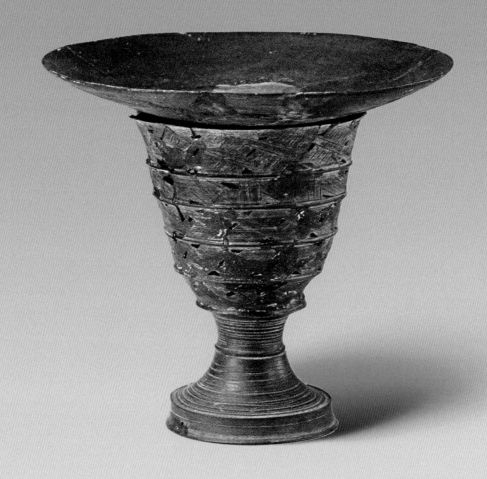

全器为两部分相套合。杯身作宽平沿，直口，深腹，圜底，套入器座内。器座状如高足杯，深腰，细柄，台形圈足。饰有纤细的凸、凹弦纹，并刻画镂空纤细的三角形、长方形、斜线形纹饰。1960 年山东省潍坊市姚官庄出土。

山东博物馆藏

The vessel is a piece of argillaceous black pottery, consisting of two nested parts, the body and the holder. The body of the cup, with a wide flat edge, a straight mouth and a round bottom, is nested into the holder, which is in the shape of a stem cup with a deep belly, a thin stem and a stand-shaped ring foot. The cup is decorated with tenuous concave-convex string designs and hollowed-out triangle, rectangle or slash motifs. It was unearthed from Yaoguanzhuang Site, Weifang City, Shandong Province, in the year 1960.

Preserved in Shandong Museum

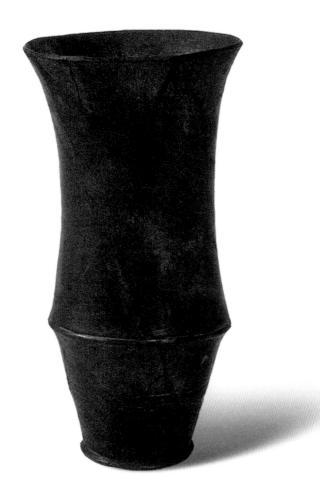

蛋壳黑陶杯

新石器时代，屈家岭文化

细泥黑陶质

口径 10 厘米，高 19 厘米

Eggshell-thin Black Pottery Cup

Qujialing Culture，Neolithic Age

Black Clay Pottery

Mouth Diameter 10 cm/ Height 19 cm

通体磨光，侈口腹，平底，矮圈足。1965 年
河南省淅川黄楝树遗址出土。

河南博物院藏

The cup, a black pottery object made of fine
slime, has a belly in the shape of a flared mouth,
a flat bottom and a short ring foot. The cup has
been polished entirely. It was unearthed from
the Huanglian Tree Site in Xichuan County,
Henan Province.

Preserved in Henan Museum

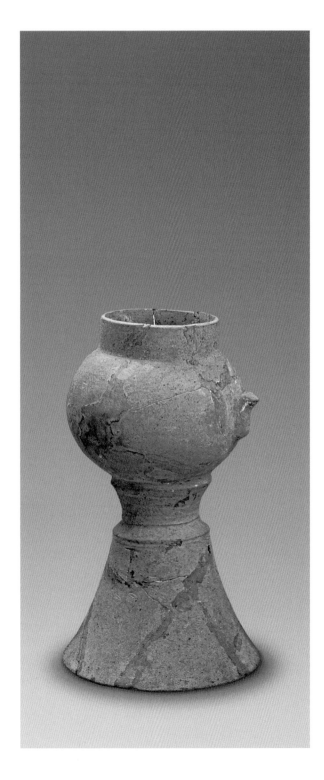

罐形陶豆

新石器时代

灰陶质

口径 13.8 厘米，通高 14 厘米

Pot-shaped Pottery "Dou" (High-stemmed Bowl)

Neolithic Age

Grey Pottery

Mouth Diameter 13.8 cm/ Height 14 cm

豆盘作折腹钵状，短唇外折，腹下部有一周垂棱。细柄高圈足，圈足表面有五组弦纹，并饰三排圆形镂孔和压印条纹。江苏省南京北阴阳营遗址 247 号墓出土。

南京市博物院藏

The "Dou", a piece of grey pottery, has an angular belly in the shape of "Bo" (bowl), a short lip bent outwards, a thin handle and a high ring foot. There is a circle of vertical ridge lines surrounding the lower part of its belly, and on the surface of the ring foot are five groups of string designs, three rows of round hollowed-out holes and embossed stripes. It was unearthed from the NO.247 Tomb of the Beiyinyangying Site in Nanjing, Jiangsu Province.

Preserved in Nanjing Municipal Museum

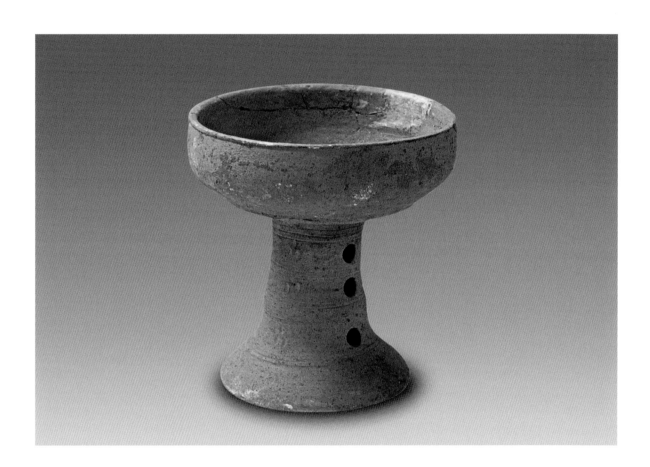

陶豆

新石器时代

泥质灰陶质

口径 5.2 厘米，高 16.7 厘米

Pottery "Dou" (High-stemmed Bowl)

Neolithic Age

Grey Clay Pottery

Mouth Diameter 5.2 cm/ Height 16.7 cm

豆盘作罐形，直口，圆鼓腹，豆把束腰，下部外撇呈喇叭状，腹部贴一小钮，腰部饰三道弦纹。器形修长匀称，器壁较薄，给人以小巧、流畅、精美之感。江苏省南京浦口营盘山遗址出土。

南京市博物馆藏

The "Dou", a piece of argillaceous grey pottery, has a straight mouth and a round swelling belly, and its upper part is in the shape of a pot. Its handle contracts in its middle part, and flares outwards in its lower part like a trumpet. There is a button and three lines of string designs on its belly. Slender and well-proportioned, the vessel exhibits features of exquisiteness, gracefulness and elegance. It was unearthed from Yingpanshan Site, Pukou District of Nanjing, Jiangsu Province.

Preserved in Nanjing Municipal Museum

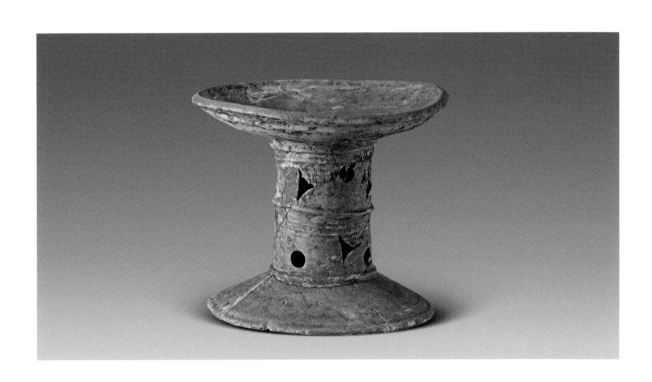

陶豆

马桥文化

陶质

口径 17 厘米，底径 16.2 厘米，高 15 厘米

遂昌县文物管理委员会藏

Pottery "Dou" (High-stemmed Bowl)

Maqiao Culture

Pottery

Mouth Diameter 17 cm/ Bottom Diameter 16.2 cm/ Height 15 cm

Preserved in Preserved in Department of Cultural Relics Coneservation of Suichang County

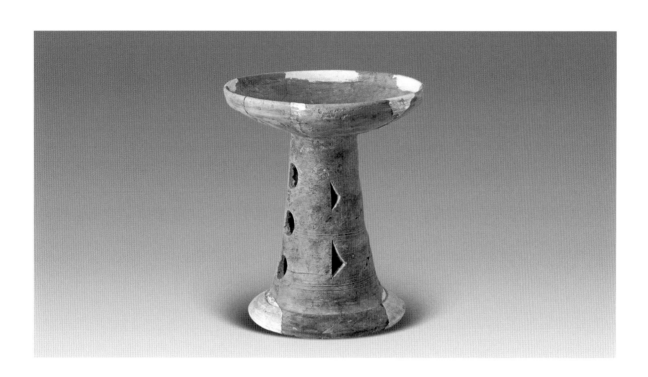

陶豆

马桥文化

陶质

口径 16.8 厘米，底径 13.8 厘米，高 19.8 厘米

遂昌县文物管理委员会藏

Pottery "Dou" (High-stemmed Bowl)

Maqiao Culture

Pottery

Diametre 16.8 cm/ Bottom Diameter 13.8 cm/ Height 19.8 cm

Preserved in Department of Cultural Relics Coneservation of Suichang County

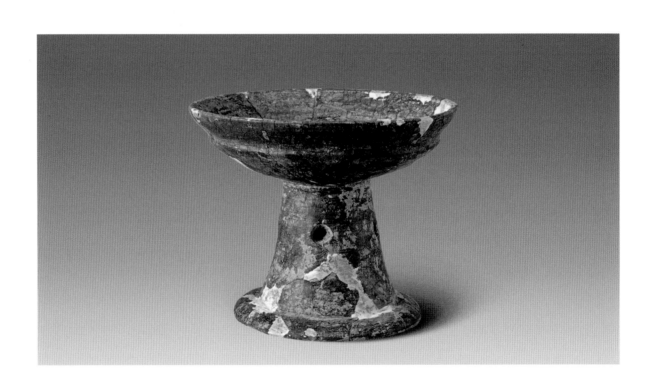

陶豆

马桥文化

泥质灰胎黑皮陶质

口径 19.4 厘米，底径 13.6 厘米，高 14.8 厘米

遂昌县文物管理委员会藏

Pottery "Dou" (High-stemmed Bowl)

Maqiao Culture

Black Clay Pottery with Grey Body

Mouth Diameter 19.4 cm/ Bottom Diameter 13.6 cm/ Height 14.8 cm

Preserved in Department of Cultural Relics Coneservation of Suichang County

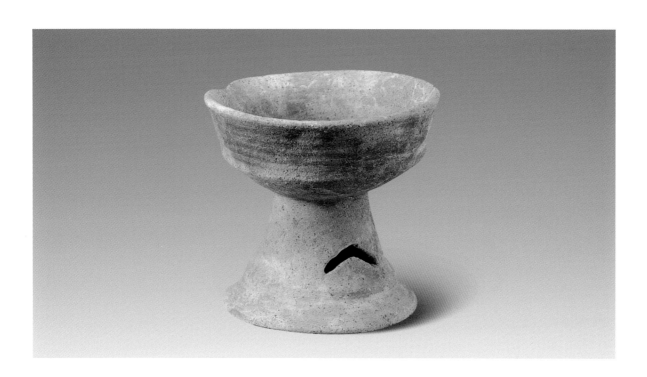

陶豆

河姆渡文化三期

陶质

口径 16.6 厘米，高 14.7 厘米

象山县文物管理委员会藏

Pottery "Dou" (High-stemmed Bowl)

Hemudu Culture Ⅲ

Pottery

Mouth Diameter 16.6 cm/ Height 14.7 cm

Preserved in Xiangshan County Administration Committee of Cultural Relics

马桥文化

泥质黑陶质

口径 17.8 厘米，底径 16.2 厘米，高 20 厘米

Maqiao Culture

Black Clay Pottery

Mouth Diameter 17.8 cm/ Bottom Diameter 16.2 cm/ Height 20 cm

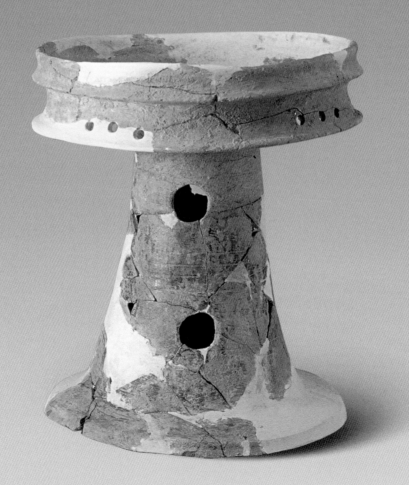

垂棱发达，垂棱上饰三组环形镂孔，一组三
个。豆把上圆形、弧边、三角形镂孔的外框
和足尖均有朱红彩。

遂昌县文物管理委员会藏

It has a wide convex hanging edge, decorated
with three sets of three ring-shaped holes. On
the handle are engraved round holes, arc holes
and triangular holes, the frames of which are
painted vermilion, so is the toe of the foot.
Preserved in Department of Cultural Relics
Coneservation of Suichang County

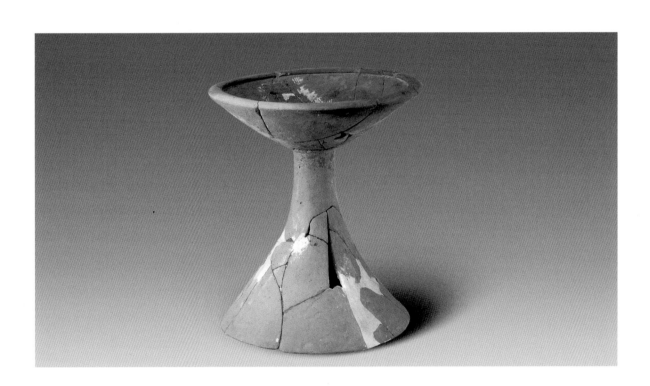

陶豆

河姆渡文化三期

陶质

口径 19.8 厘米，高 23.3 厘米

浙江省文物考古研究所藏

Pottery "Dou" (High-stemmed Bowl)

Hemudu Culture Ⅲ

Pottery

Mouth Diameter 19.8 cm/ Height 23.3 cm

Preserved in Institute of Cultural Relics and Archaeology of Zhejiang Province

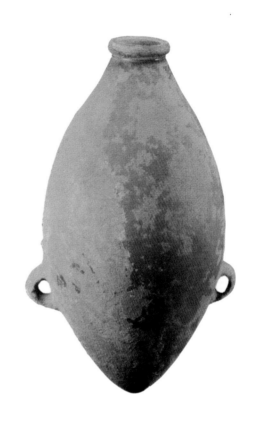

尖底瓶

新石器时代，仰韶文化

陶质

口外径 5.7 厘米，腹围 156.5 厘米，高 36.5 厘米

取水器。1970 年陕西渭南征集。

陕西医史博物馆藏

Bottle with Pointed Bottom

Yangshao Culture, Neolithic Age

Pottery

Outer Mouth Diameter 5.7 cm/ Belly Perimeter 156.5 cm/ Height 36.5 cm

This bottle was used to fetch water and collected from Weinan County, Shaanxi Province, in the year 1970.

Preserved in Shaanxi Museum of Medical History

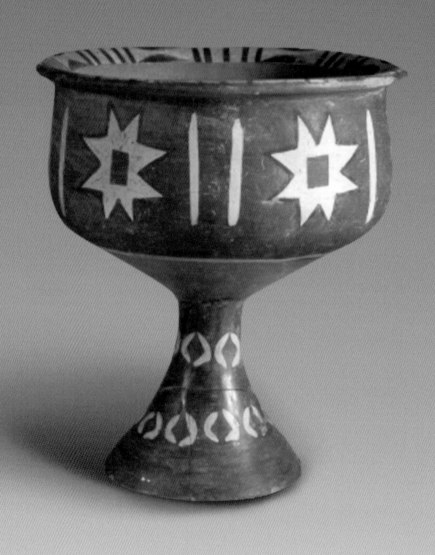

八角星纹彩陶豆

新石器时代，大汶口文化

泥质红陶质

口径 26 厘米，足径 14.5 厘米，高 29.5 厘米

施红色陶衣。口沿外折，深腹，下为喇叭形足。口沿以白彩绘地，赭彩绘直线纹及三角纹；腹部用白彩绘方形空心八角纹，并用黑彩描边；足上用赭彩绘地，白彩绘对弧线纹。八角星纹图案在大汶口文化中颇富特色。食器。1974 年山东省泰安市大汶口村出土。

山东省文物考古研究所藏

Painted Pottery "Dou" (High-stemmed Bowl) with Octagonal Star Designs

Dawenkou Culture, Neolithic Age

Red Clay Pottery

Mouth Diameter 26 cm/ Foot Diametre 14.5 cm/ Height 29.5 cm

This vessel, coated with red colour, has an everted mouth-rim, a deep belly and a flared foot. Its mouth-rim is painted white and decorated with ochre straight stripes and triangles, while its belly is embellished with hollowed-out octagonal stars in white, which are framed with black lines. Its foot is painted ochre and decorated with white arc lines. The design of octagonal stars is a typical feature of Dawenkou Culture. This vessel was used as a food container, and in the year 1974 it was unearthed in Dawenkou Village of Taian, Shandong Province.

Preserved in Institute of Cultural Relics and Archaeology of Shandong Drovince

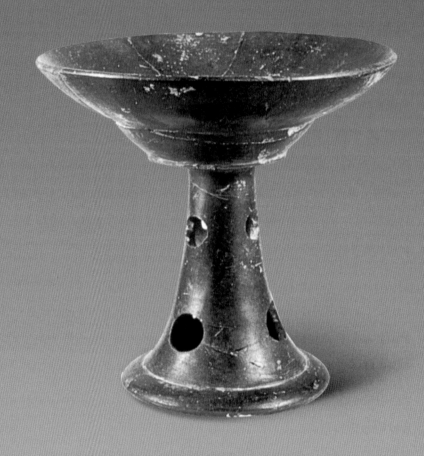

黑陶高柄豆

新石器时代晚期，庙底沟文化二期（前 3000—前 2700）

黑陶质

口径 23.5 厘米，高 22.2 厘米

Black Pottery "Dou" (High-stemmed Bowl)

Miaodigou Culture Ⅱ (3000 B.C.–2700 B.C.), Late Neolithic Age

Black Pottery

Mouth Diameter 23.5 cm/ Height 22.2 cm

加有高底座的浅盘。胎体是细致的泥质灰陶，造型不失生动；表皮经过工艺处理呈黑色的"黑皮陶"，外观黑而亮泽，庄重典雅。盛放食品的器具。河南省洛阳市王湾遗址出土。

北京大学赛克勒考古与艺术博物馆藏

This "Dou" has a shallow plate on a tall base, and its body is made of fine argillaceous grey pottery. The surface of the vessel, after being processed, shows the feature of "Hei Pi Tao" (pottery with a black coating) with black lustre. It is vivid and elegant in style and served well as a food container. It was unearthed from Wangwan Site in Luoyang, Henan Province. Preserved in Arthur M. Sackler Museum of Art and Archaeology at Peking University

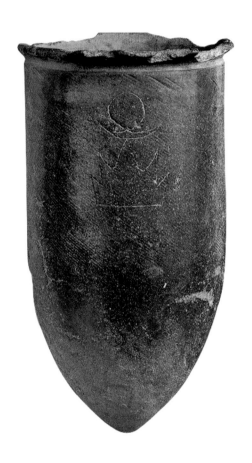

灰陶尊

新石器时代，大汶口文化

夹砂灰陶质

口径 29.5 厘米，高 57.5 厘米

Grey Pottery "Zun" (Wine Vessel)

Dawenkou Culture，Neolithic Age

Grey Sandy Pottery

Mouth Diameter 29.5 cm/ Height 57.5 cm

胎体特别厚重。大口，深腹，尖底。属于盛
酒的祭器。1961 年山东省莒县陵阳河出土。

莒州博物馆藏

The vessel, with a very thick body, a big
mouth, a deep belly and a pointed bottom,
is a sacrificial utensil to serve wine. It was
unearthed from Lingyang River in Juxian
County, Shandong Province, in the year 1961.
Preserved in Juzhou Museum

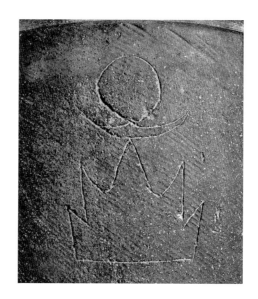

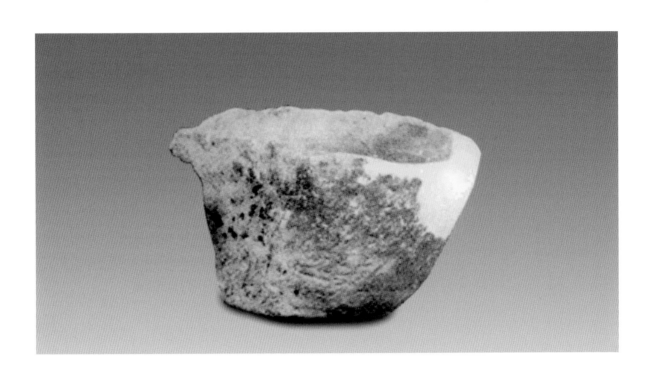

匜

新石器时代，齐家文化

灰陶质

口径 13.7 厘米，底径 8.9 厘米，高 9 厘米

盛水盥洗用具。青海柳湾出土。

青海柳湾彩陶博物馆藏

"Yi" (Gourd-shaped Ladle)

Qijia Culture, Neolithic Age

Grey Pottery

Mouth Diameter 13.7 cm/ Bottom Diameter 8.9 cm/
Height 9 cm

This vessel was used to hold water for face or hand
washing. It was unearthed in Liuwan tomb in Qinghai
Province.

Preserved in Liuwan Painted Pottery Museum,
Qinghai Province

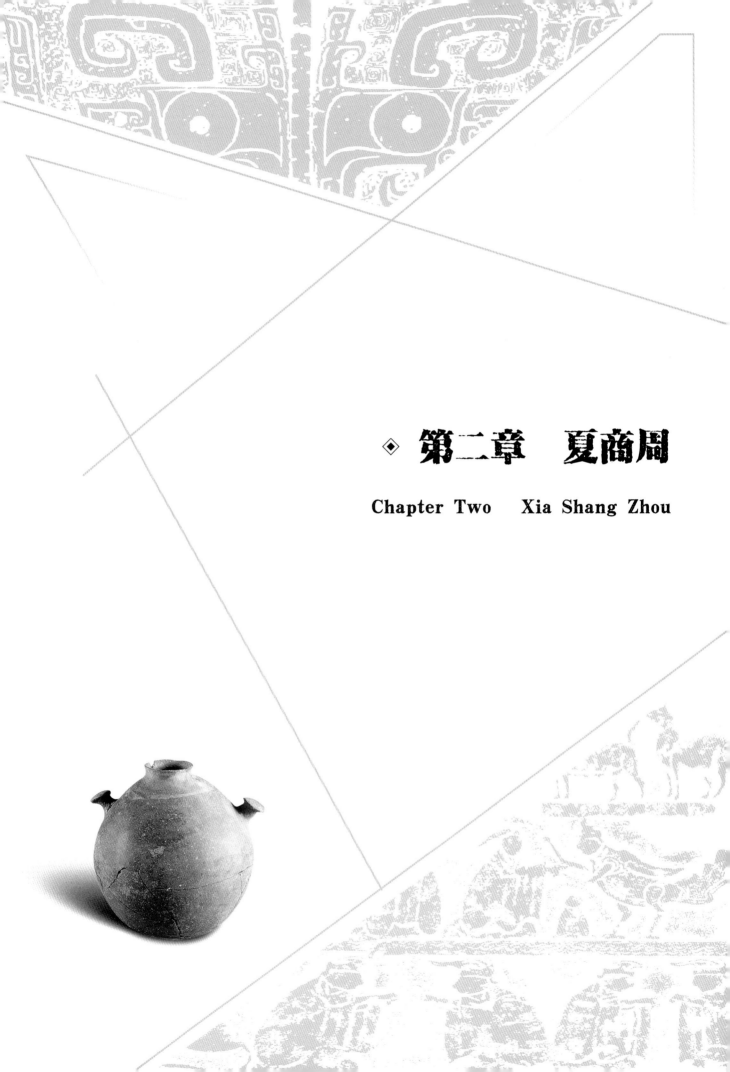

◇ 第二章　夏商周

Chapter Two　Xia Shang Zhou

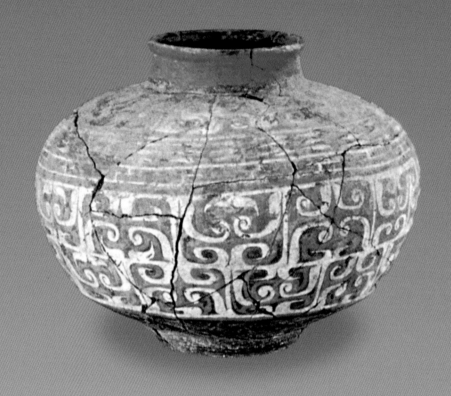

彩绘陶罐

夏家店下层文化（前 21 世纪—前 16 世纪）

陶质

口径 9.4 厘米，腹径 25 厘米，底径 8.2 厘米，高 19 厘米

Painted Pottery Pot

Lower Xiajiadian Culture (21st Century B.C. —16th Century B.C.)

Pottery

Mouth Diameter 9.4 cm/ Belly Diametre 25 cm/ Bottom Diameter 8.2 cm/ Height 19 cm

该器造型饱满匀称。罐身上在黑色底衬上用红白二色绘出二方连续的多单元繁缛几何纹，这在中原地区同时代的陶器中绝难见到，但它的几何图案的构图却表明了与中原腹地古代文化的姻亲关系。常用盛贮器。内蒙古赤峰市大甸子遗址出土。

北京大学赛克勒考古与艺术博物馆藏

The pot is well-balanced and plump-shaped. On the black body are painted multi-units of consecutive geometric patterns with red and white pigments, which are rarely seen among the pottery vessels of the contemporary period in the central China. However, the design of the geometric patterns shows relationship by affinity in the ancient culture of the central China. It was often used for storage. It was unearthed from Dadianzi Site in Chifeng, Inner Mongolia.

Preserved in Arthur M. Sackler Museum of Art and Archaeology at Peking University

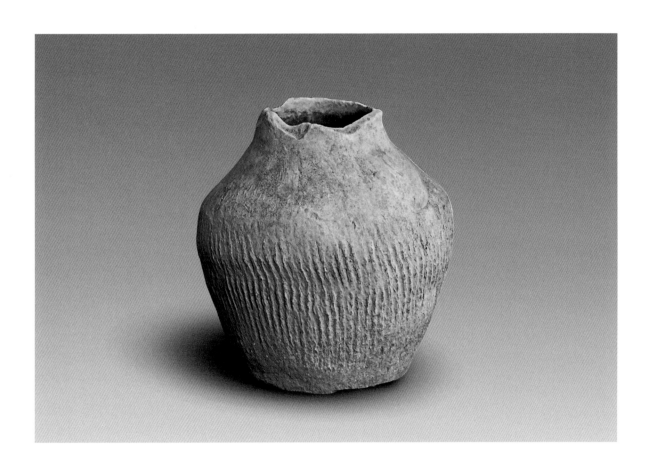

陶罐

西周

陶质

口径 7 厘米，底径 9 厘米，高 14 厘米，重 600 克

Pottery Pot

Western Zhou Dynasty

Pottery

Mouth Diameter 7 cm/ Bottom Diameter 9 cm/ Height 14 cm/ Weight 600 g

溜肩，斜腹，平底，腹部粗绳纹。盛贮器，口沿全残。陕西省白水县洞陇上征集。

陕西医史博物馆藏

The pot has a sloping shoulder, an oblique belly with thick cord patterns on the surface and a flat bottom. The storage pot, with its mouth rim totally damaged, was collected from Donglongshang in Baishui County, Shaanxi Province.

Preserved in Shaanxi Museum of Medical History

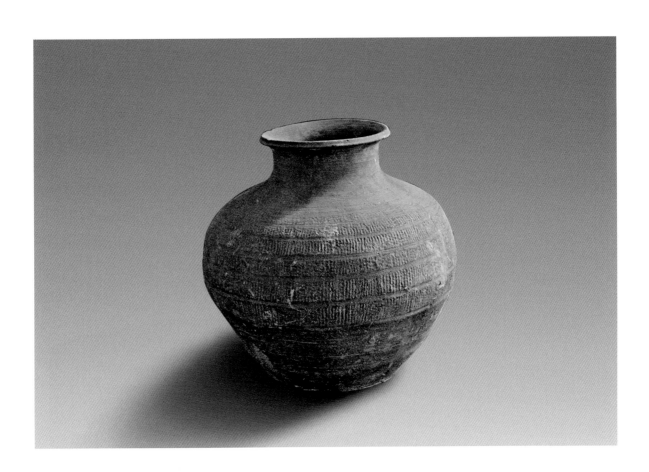

绳纹灰陶罐

西周

陶质

口径 8.8 厘米，底径 10.2 厘米，通高 16 厘米，重 850 克

Grey Pottery Pot with Rope Design

Western Zhou Dynasty

Pottery

Mouth Diameter 8.8 cm/ Bottom Diameter 10.2 cm/ Height 16 cm/ Weight 850 g

灰色，绳纹，侈口，鼓腹，平底。肩上有铭文。
盛贮器，生活用器物。完整无损。

陕西医史博物馆藏

The pottery pot is grey and decorated with rope designs. It has a flared mouth, a swelling belly, and a flat bottom. Inscriptions can be seen on the shoulder. The pot, perfectly preserved, is a piece of household ware for storage.

Preserved in Shaanxi Museum of Medical History

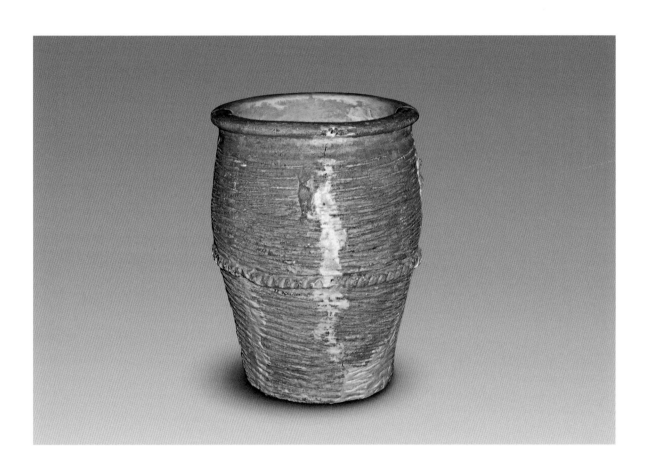

陶罐

西周

陶质

口径 15.5 厘米，底径 11.5 厘米，通高 21 厘米，重 1550 克

Pottery Pot

Western Zhou Dynasty

Pottery

Mouth Diameter 15.5 cm/ Bottom Diameter 11.5 cm/ Height 21 cm/ Weight 1,550 g

平口沿，直斜腹，腹中间一道凸棱纹筐纹，平底。盛贮器。2/3 处有修补。陕西省西安市征集。

陕西医史博物馆藏

The pot, with a flat rim, a straight sloping belly, and a flat bottom, was used for storage. On the middle of its belly is a ridge line in the shape of a basketwork. Two-thirds of the pot has been restored. It was collected from Xi'an, Shaanxi Province.

Preserved in Shaanxi Museum of Medical History

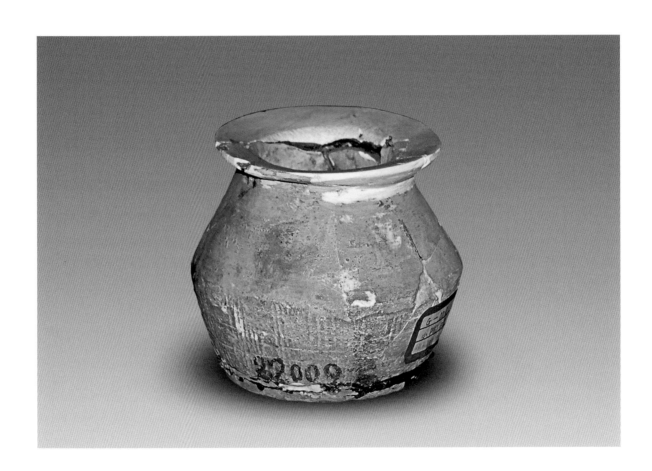

陶罐

西周

红陶质

口径 7.8 厘米，底径 7.3 厘米，通高 8 厘米，重 380 克

Pottery Pot

Western Zhou Dynasty

Red Pottery

Mouth Diameter 7.8 cm/ Bottom Diameter 7.3 cm/ Height 8 cm/ Weight 380 g

口沿外敞，折肩，平底。盛贮器。周身有修补。

陕西省兴平市征集。

陕西医史博物馆藏

With a flared mouth, an angular shoulder and
a flat bottom, the pot was used for storage.
The body of the pot has been repaired. It
was collected from Xingping City, Shaanxi
Province.

Preserved in Shaanxi Museum of Medical History

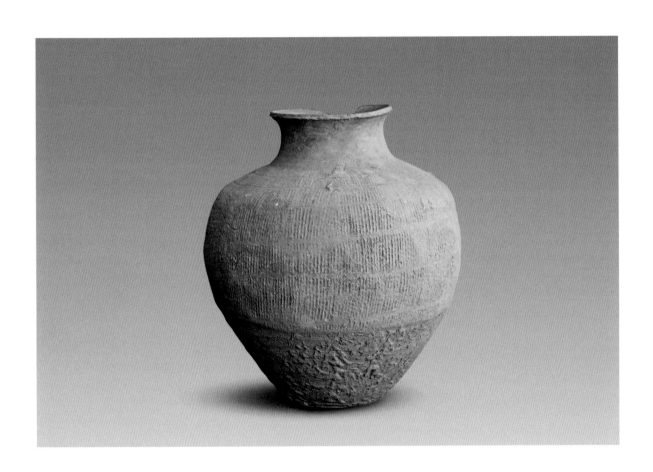

陶罐

西周

灰陶质

口径 9.8 厘米，底径 8.6 厘米，高 23 厘米，重 1500 克

Pottery Pot

Western Zhou Dynasty

Grey Pottery

Mouth Diameter 9.8 cm/ Bottom Diameter 8.6 cm/ Height 23 cm/ Weight 1,500 g

侈口，平肩，直腹，平底。上腹为绳纹。盛贮器。
口沿残。陕西省澄城县征集。

陕西医史博物馆藏

The pot, with a flared mouth, a flat shoulder, a straight belly, and a flat bottom, was used for storage. Its upper belly is decorated with cord patterns. The mouth rim is damaged. It was collected from Chengcheng County, Shaanxi Province.

Preserved in Shaanxi Museum of Medical History

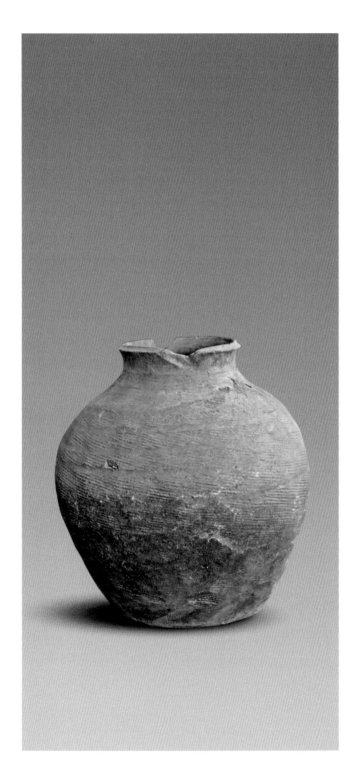

陶罐

西周

灰陶质

口径 9.5 厘米，底径 12 厘米，高 21 厘米，
重 1550 克

Pottery Pot

Western Zhou Dynasty

Grey Pottery

Mouth Diameter 9.5 cm/ Bottom Diameter

12 cm/ Height 21 cm/ Weight 1,550 g

侈口，溜肩，圆腹，平底。上腹部为绳纹。

盛贮器。口沿残。陕西省澄城县征集。

陕西医史博物馆藏

With a flared mouth, a sloping shoulder, a round belly and a flat bottom, the pot was used for storage. Cord patterns can be seen on the upper belly. Its mouth rim was damaged. It was collected from Chengcheng County in Shaanxi Province.

Preserved in Shaanxi Museum of Medical History

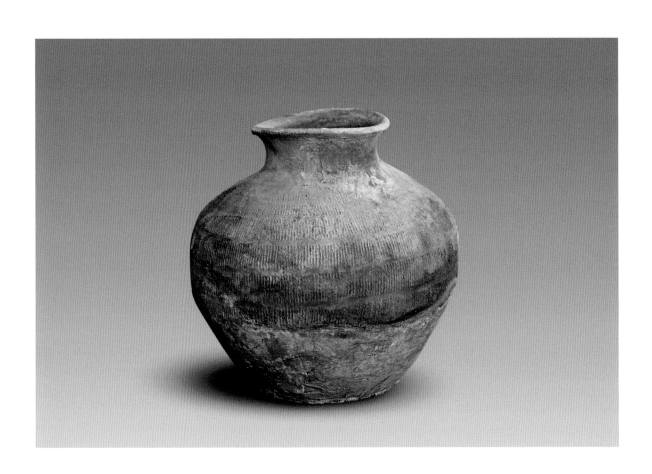

陶罐

西周

陶质

口径 9.8 厘米，底径 10.8 厘米，高 19.6 厘米，重 1500 克

Pottery Pot

Western Zhou Dynasty

Pottery

Mouth Diameter 9.8 cm/ Bottom Diameter 10.8 cm/ Height 19.6 cm/ Weight 1,550 g

侈口，溜肩，圆腹，平底。上腹部为绳纹。
盛贮器。完整无损。陕西省澄城县征集。

陕西医史博物馆藏

With a flared mouth, a sloping shoulder, a round belly and a flat bottom, the pot was used for storage. Its upper belly is decorated with cord patterns. It is well preserved and was collected from Chengcheng County in Shaanxi Province. Preserved in Shaanxi Museum of Medical History

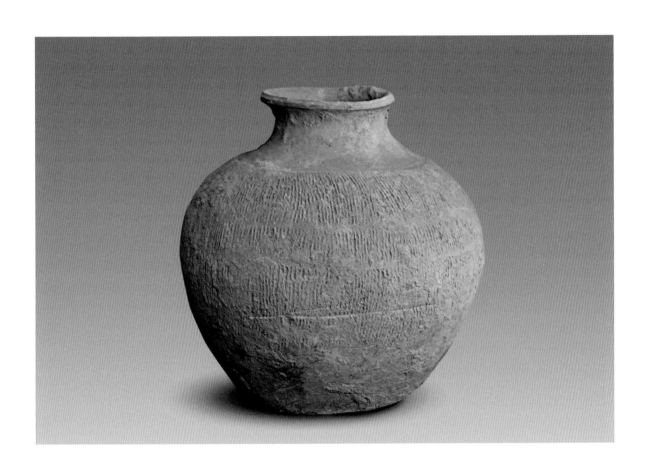

陶罐

西周

灰陶质

口径 10.03 厘米，底径 14.8 厘米，高 13.3 厘米，重 1950 克

Pottery Pot

Western Zhou Dynasty

Grey Pottery

Mouth Diameter 10.03 cm/ Bottom Diameter 14.8 cm/ Height 13.3 cm/ Weight 1,950 g

侈口，圆肩，圆腹，平底。上腹部为绳纹。

盛贮器，完整无损。陕西省澄城县征集。

陕西医史博物馆藏

With a flared mouth, a round shoulder, a round belly and a flat bottom, the pot was used for storage. Its upper belly is decorated with cord patterns. The pot, well preserved, was collected from Chengcheng County, Shaanxi Province.

Preserved in Shaanxi Museum of Medical History

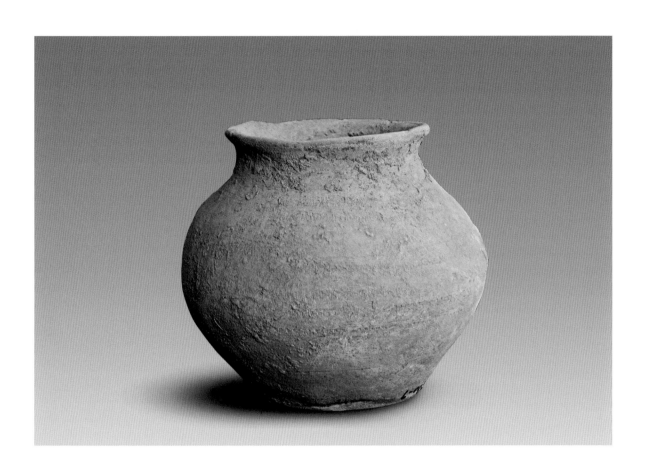

陶罐

西周

灰陶质

口径 13.5 厘米，底径 12.5 厘米，高 18.2 厘米，重 1500 克

Pottery Pot

Western Zhou Dynasty

Grey Pottery

Mouth Diameter 13.5 cm/ Bottom Diameter 12.5 cm/ Height 18.2 cm/ Weight 1,500 g

口沿不规则，侈口，圆腹，平底。通体为篦纹。

盛贮器。完整无损。陕西省澄城县征集。

陕西医史博物馆藏

The pot, with a flared mouth, the rim of which
is irregular, a round belly and a flat bottom, was
used for storage. The entire body of the pot is
decorated with fine-toothed comb designs and
is perfectly preserved. It was collected from
Chengcheng County in Shaanxi Province.
Preserved in Shaanxi Museum of Medical History

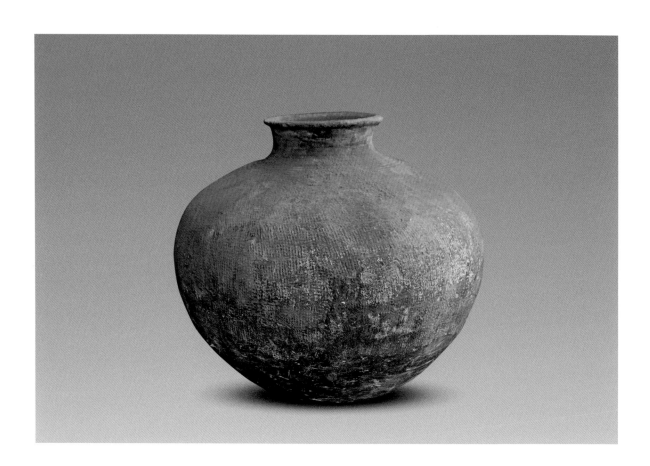

陶罐

西周

灰陶质

口径 10.06 厘米，底径 13.3 厘米，高 24.3 厘米，重 2650 克

Pottery Pot

Western Zhou Dynasty

Grey Pottery

Mouth Diameter 10.06 cm/ Bottom Diameter 13.3 cm/ Height 24.3 cm/ Weight 2,650 g

侈口，圆腹，平底。肩部数道弦纹，上腹部
为细绳纹。盛贮器。完整无损。陕西省澄城
县征集。

陕西医史博物馆藏

The pot has a flared mouth, a round belly, and
a flat bottom. Its shoulder is decorated with
several rings of string patterns while its upper
belly is embellished with cord patterns. It was
used for storage and is perfectly preserved.
It was collected from Chengcheng County in
Shaanxi Province.

Preserved in Shaanxi Museum of Medical History

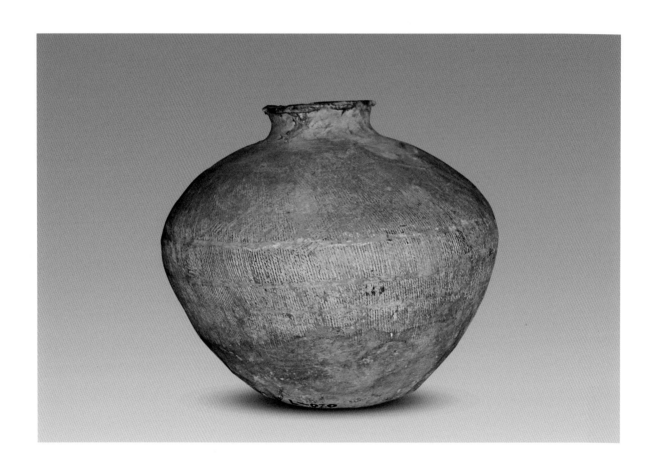

绳纹陶罐

西周

灰陶质

口径 11 厘米，底径 16 厘米，高 27.2 厘米，重 3400 克

Pottery Pot with Rope Design

Western Zhou Dynasty

Grey Pottery

Mouth Diameter 11 cm/ Bottom Diameter 16 cm/ Height 27.2 cm/ Weight 3,400 g

唇口，斜肩，圆腹，平底。腹上部有细绳纹。

生活器具。口沿残。陕西省澄城县征集。

陕西医史博物馆藏

The pot has a lip-shaped mouth-rim, a sloping shoulder, a round belly, and a flat bottom. Its upper belly is decorated with cord patterns. Its mouth rim was damaged. It was a piece of household ware and collected from Chengcheng County in Shaanxi Province. Preserved in Shaanxi Museum of Medical History

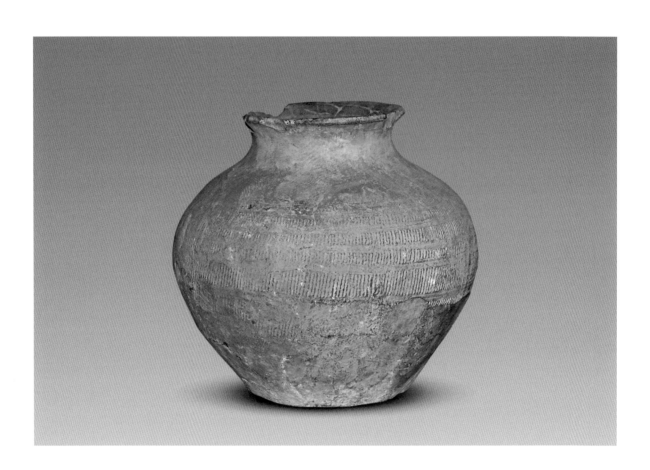

陶罐

西周

灰陶质

口径 11.5 厘米，底径 11 厘米，高 19.8 厘米，重 1800 克

Pottery Pot

Western Zhou Dynasty

Grey Pottery

Mouth Diameter 11.5 cm/ Bottom Diameter 11 cm/ Height 19.8 cm/ Weight 1,800 g

侈口，圆腹，平底。腹部有绳纹。盛贮器。
口沿残。陕西省澄城县征集。

陕西医史博物馆藏

The pot has a flared mouth, a round belly, and a flat bottom. Its mouth rim is damaged, and its belly is decorated with cord patterns. It was used for storage and collected from Chengcheng County, Shaanxi Province.

Preserved in Shaanxi Museum of Medical History

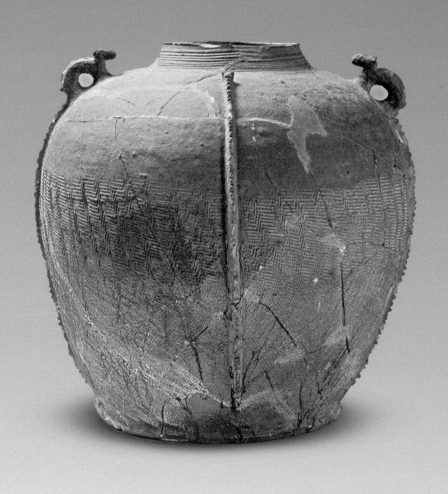

兽耳印纹硬陶罐

西周

陶质

口径 11.4 厘米，底径 21.4 厘米，高 34 厘米

口沿内敛，溜肩，下腹内收，平底。口沿下有数道细弦纹，肩部各塑一兽耳，腹身堆贴四条扉棱，其中两条与兽耳相连，并饰有曲折纹与回纹相结合的几何纹饰。此器质地坚硬，造型端庄，形制独特，具有地方特色。江苏省南京市溧水区乌山镇岗沿山西周墓出土。

镇江博物馆藏

Stamped Ornamentation Pottery Pot with Double Beast-shaped Ears

Western Zhou Dynasty

Pottery

Mouth Diameter 11.4 cm/ Bottom Diameter 21.4 cm/ Height 34 cm

The jar has a contracted mouth, a sloping shoulder and a flat bottom. There are several rings of thin string patterns just below the mouth rim and a pair of beast-shaped ears on the shoulder. On the belly are moulded four convex lines, two of which are connected to the ears. The belly is also decorated with geometric patterns, a combination of zigzag patterns and rectangular spiral patterns. The hard texture, elegant design, and the unique shape show the local features. It was unearthed from the tomb of the Western Zhou Dynasty in Gangyan Mountain, Wushan Town, Lishui District, Nanjing City, Jiangsu Province.

Preserved in Zhenjiang Museum

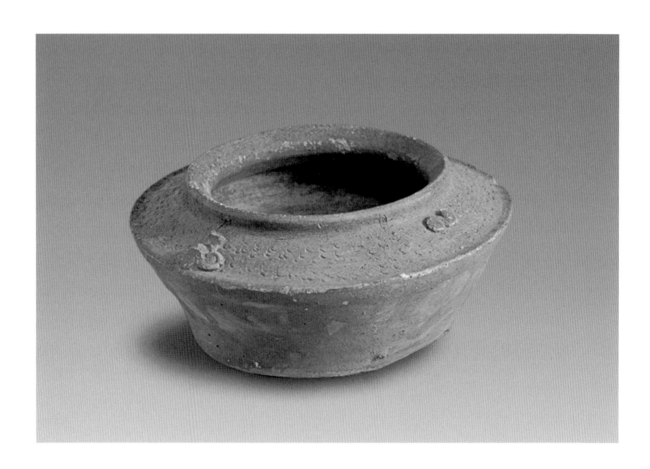

着黑硬陶罐

西周晚期

陶质

口径 9.6 厘米，底径 10 厘米，高 6.1 厘米

Hard Pottery Pot Painted in Black

Late Western Zhou Dynasty

Pottery

Mouth Diameter 9.6 cm/ Bottom Diameter 10 cm/ Height 6.1 cm

此器通体着有黑色涂层，黑层无光亮感，与
瓷釉有别。

浙江省文物考古研究所藏

The whole body is painted black without lustre,
different from porcelain glaze.
Preserved in Institute of Cultural Relics and
Archaeology of Zhejiang Province

青釉原始瓷罐

东周

瓷质

口径 11.5 厘米，高 17.5 厘米

Eastern Zhou Dynasty

Porcelain

Mouth Diameter 11.5 cm/ Height 17.5 cm

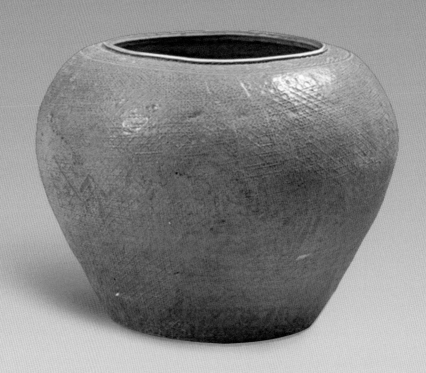

胎呈青灰色，满施黄绿色釉。直口，宽肩，圆腹，平底。刻画水波纹，外壁拍印细太阳纹，纹饰精美，制作规整，属早期瓷器产品。该藏是研究中国早期瓷器发展和吴越文化的珍贵资料。

南京博物院藏

The body of the pot is caesious and is coated with yellowish-green glaze. It has a straight mouth, a broad shoulder, a round belly and a flat bottom. It is incised with ripple designs and exquisite thin swirl marks, arranged in regular order. It is a piece of early porcelain ware in Chinese history, extremely precious for the research of the development of the early Chinese porcelain and the Wuyue Culture.

Preserved in Nanjing Museum

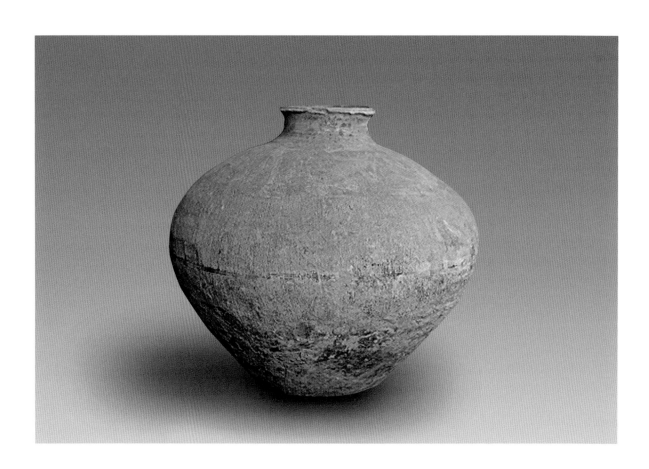

陶罐

周

灰陶质

口径 11 厘米，底径 15 厘米，高 31.5 厘米，重 4150 克

Pottery Jar

Zhou Dynasty

Grey Pottery

Mouth Diameter 11 cm/ Bottom Diameter 15 cm/ Height 31.5 cm/ Weight 4,150 g

圆唇，溜肩，圆腹，平底。肩腹部饰细绳纹，腹下部素面。盛贮器。完整无损。

陕西医史博物馆藏

The jar has a round lip, a sloping shoulder, a globular belly and a flat bottom, with fine string patterns around the shoulder and on the upper belly, but looks plain on the lower belly. This grey pottery ware, well preserved, was used as a container.

Preserved in Shaanxi Museum of Medical History

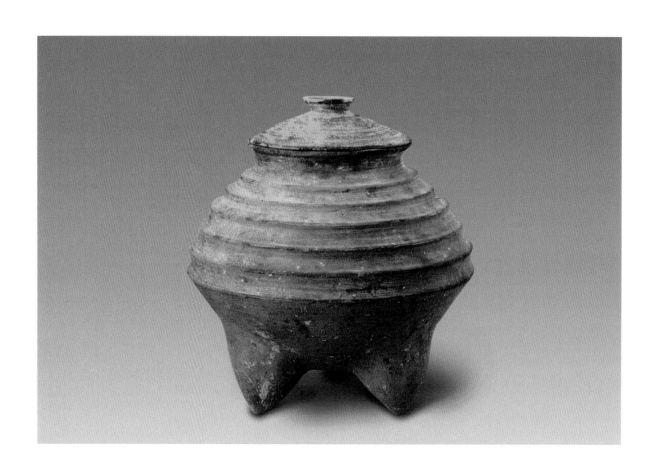

灰陶折腹鼎

西周中期 (前 950—前 850)

灰陶质

最大腹径 23.2 厘米，高 24 厘米

Grey Pottery "Ding" (Tripod) with Angular Belly

Mid Western Zhou Dynasty (950 B.C.‒850 B.C.)

Grey Pottery

Maximum Belly Diametre 23.2 cm/ Height 24 cm

鼎与鬲的主要区别在于三足的实与空，后世文献中便有"鬲是空足之鼎"之说。此件陶炊器总体造型似一带有三只矮空足的小口瓮，足虽空但主要盛贮空间仍在腹部，故仍以鼎称之，或谓之为"瓮鼎"。空足鼎可视为鼎中的异型。山西省曲沃县晋国墓地出土。

北京大学赛克勒考古与艺术博物馆藏

The major difference between "Ding" and "Li" is that the legs are solid for "Ding" but hollow for "Li". As is recorded in the historical documents, "Li is a Ding with hollow legs". This pottery cooking utensil is in the shape of an urn with a small mouth and three short hollow legs. Despite hollow legs, the belly serves as the main containing space, justifying the name "Ding", or "Wong Ding" (urn-shaped tripod). The hollow-legged "Ding" is uncommon compared with normal ones. It was unearthed in a tomb of Jin State in the Spring-Autumn Period, Quwo County, Shanxi Province.

Preserved in Arthur M. Sackler Museum of Art and Archaeology at Peking University

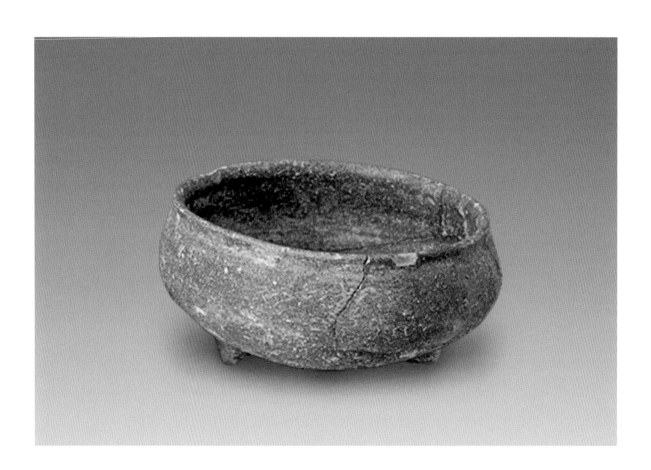

着黑硬陶鼎

西周晚期

陶质

口径 13.2 厘米，通高 6.6 厘米

Black Hard Pottery "Ding" (Tripod)

Late Western Zhou Dynasty

Pottery

Mouth Diameter 13.2 cm/ Height 6.6 cm

内、外壁均施无光泽的黑色涂层，并可见涂
刷黑层时的流挂现象。

瑞安博物馆藏

Both the interior and exterior of the tripod
are covered by unpolished black coating. The
sagging left on the surface during the painting
process remains noticeable.
Preserved in Rui'an Museum

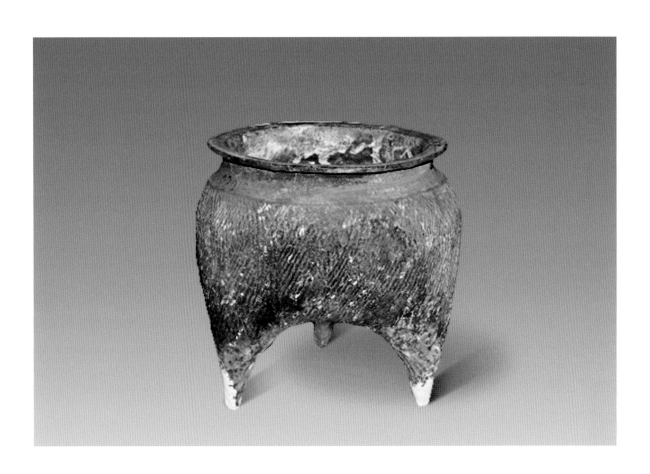

陶鬲

商

灰陶质

口径 16 厘米，通高 17.5 厘米，重 1050 克

Pottery "Li" (Cauldron)

Shang Dynasty

Grey Pottery

Mouth Diameter 16 cm/ Height 17.5 cm/ Weight 1,050 g

平口沿，三乳足。周身饰粗绳纹。炊器。两足有修补。陕西省鄠邑区征集。

陕西医史博物馆藏

This "Li" has a flat mouth and three breast-shaped legs, with heavy string patterns all over the belly. This grey pottery ware was used as a cooking utensil. Two of the three legs were repaired. It was collected from Huyi District, Shaanxi province.

Preserved in Shaanxi Museum of Medical History

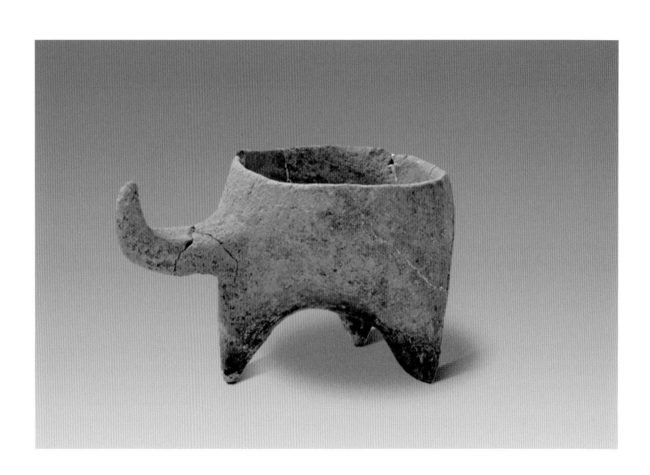

陶鬲

商周

夹砂陶质

Pottery "Li" (Cauldron)

Shang and Zhou Dynasties

Sandy Pottery

商周时代的炊煮用器。下部有烟炱痕，属秦淮河流域的湖熟文化遗存。其基本造型受到黄河流域文化的影响，但角状把手却具备江南特色，反映出南北文化兼容的特征，是研究商周时代南京地方文化面貌的典型材料之一。

南京博物院藏

This "Li" was a cooking utensil in Shang and Zhou Dynasties. Soot marks can be found at the lower body of this cultural relic of Hu-shu Culture in Qinhuai River Basin. The basic design has been affected by the culture of the Yellow River Basin, while the hornlike handle reflects the characteristics of South China, indicating the combination of South and North civilizations. Therefore, this is a typical material for studying the regional culture in Nanjing during Shang and Zhou Dynasties.

Preserved in Nanjing Museum

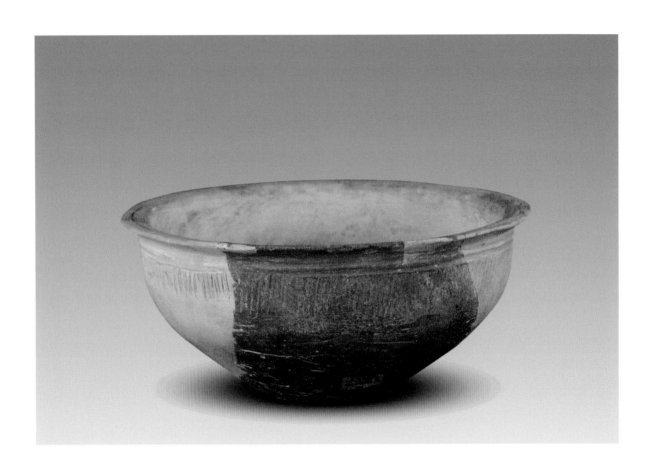

陶盆

周

陶质

口径 23 厘米，底径 8 厘米，通高 9.5 厘米，重 600 克

Pottery Basin

Zhou Dynasty

Pottery

Mouth Diameter 23 cm/ Bottom Diameter 8 cm/ Height 9.5 cm/ Weight 600 g

敞口，平口沿，折腹，平底。上腹有绳纹。食器。
三分之二残，已修补。陕西历史博物馆调拨。

陕西医史博物馆藏

The basin has a flaring mouth, a flattened mouth
rim, an angular belly and a flat bottom, with
string patterns around the upper belly. It served
as a food container, with two thirds of which
being restored. The basin was allocated from
Shaanxi History Museum.

Preserved in Shaanxi Museum of Medical History

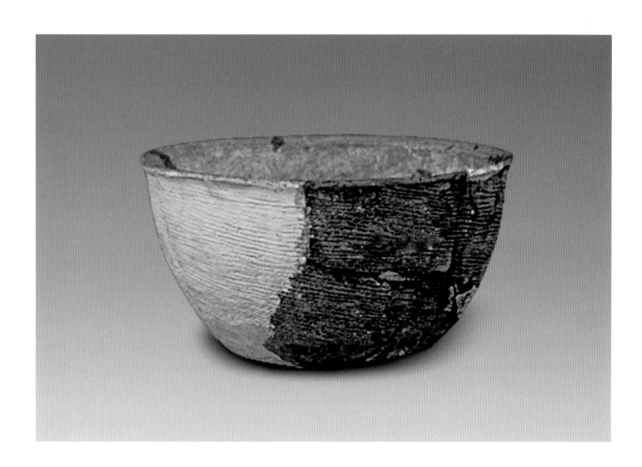

陶盆

周

陶质

口径 24.5 厘米，底径 13.5 厘米，通高 12.4 厘米，重 110 克

Pottery Basin

Zhou Dynasty

Pottery

Mouth Diameter 24.5 cm/ Bottom Diameter 13.5 cm/ Height 12.4 cm/ Weight 110 g

侈口，圆腹，平底。周身饰绳纹。食器。三分之二残，已修补。陕西历史博物馆调拨。

陕西医史博物馆藏

The basin has a wide flared mouth, a round belly and a flat bottom, with string pattern all over the body. It is a food container, with two thirds of which being restored. The basin was allocated from Shaanxi History Museum.

Preserved in Shaanxi Museum of Medical History

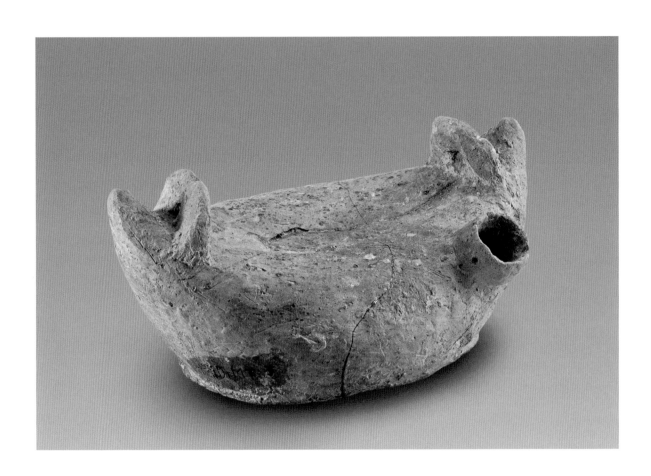

硬陶船形壶

西周早期

陶质

长 22.6 厘米，宽 14 厘米，高 9.7 厘米

Hard Pottery Boat-shaped Pot

Early Western Zhou Dynasty

Pottery

Length 22.6 cm/ Width 14 cm/ Height 9.7 cm

素面硬陶器。扁腹大平底，平面呈船形，两端呈尖状上翘，并各有一圆形竖耳，中有耳孔可穿绳。一侧设有圆形短流。形制特殊，为少见之物。1989 年浙江省长兴县石狮村土墩墓出土。

浙江省文物考古研究所藏

The plain hard pottery pot has a flat belly and a flat bottom. The plane of the body is in the shape of a boat, with both pointed ends upward. At each of the two ends, there is a round prick ear respectively, through which a cord can get. A short spout in round shape can be found on one side. The special design has rarely been seen. It was unearthed at the mound tomb in Shishi Village, Changxing County, Zhejiang Province, in the year 1989.

Preserved in Institute of Cultural Relics and Archaeology of Zhejiang Province

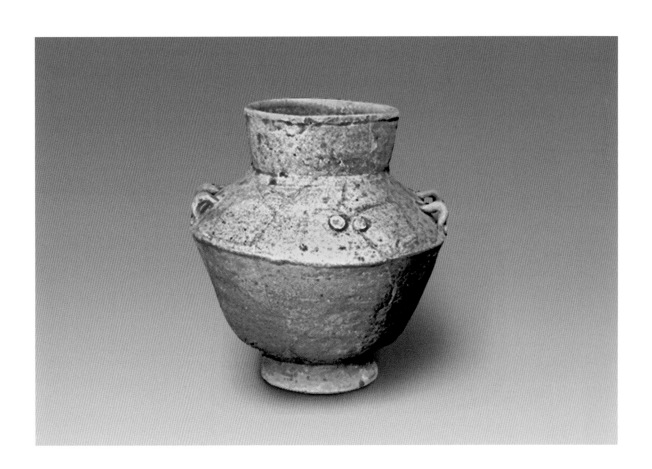

青瓷壶

西周

瓷质

高 22 厘米

Celadon Pot

Western Zhou Dynasty

Porcelain

Height 22 cm

青黄釉。我国存世最早的青瓷器具，可用于
盛酒或水。陕西扶风周原遗址出土。

宝鸡市周原博物馆藏

This greenish-yellow-glazed pot is the earliest
celadon pot existed in the world. It served as
a wine or water vessel. It was unearthed from
Zhouyuan Site in Fufeng County, Shaanxi
Province.

Preserved in Zhouyuan Museum, Baoji City

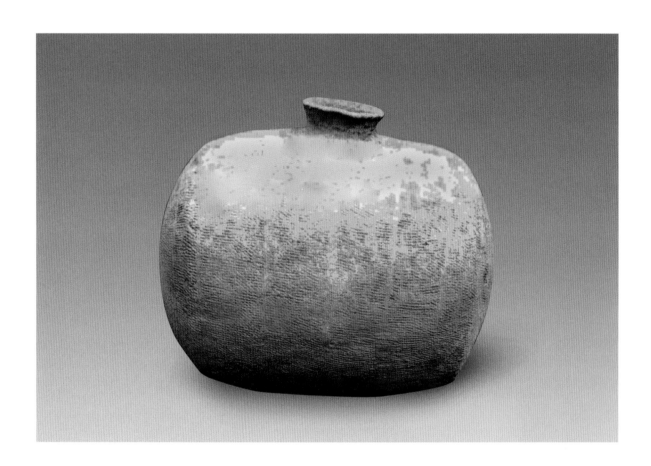

鸭蛋壶

西周

灰陶质

口径 14.7 厘米，颈高 4.6 厘米，长 59.5 厘米，通高 55.5 厘米

Duckegg-shaped Pot

Western Zhou Dynasty

Grey Pottery

Mouth Diameter 14.7 cm/ Neck Height 4.6 cm/ Length 59.5 cm/ Height 55.5 cm

鸭蛋形。容器。陕西扶风周原遗址出土。

宝鸡市周原博物馆藏

The duckegg-shaped pot served as a container,
and was unearthed from Zhouyuan Site, Fufeng
County, Shaanxi Province.
Preserved in Zhouyuan Museum, Baoji City

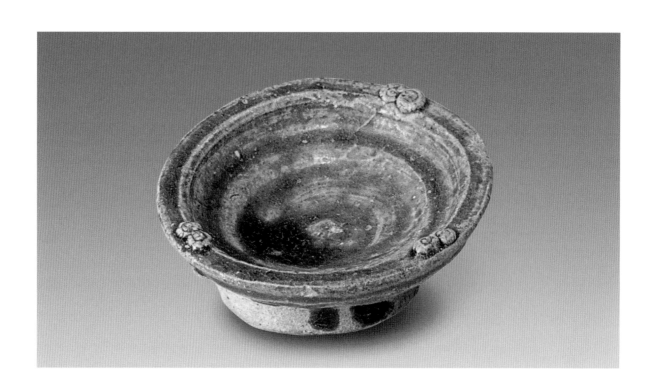

原始青瓷碟

西周晚期

瓷质

口径 7.4 厘米，底径 4.6 厘米，高 2.6 厘米

瑞安博物馆藏

Primitive Celadon Plate

Late Western Zhou Dynasty

Porcelain

Mouth Diameter 7.4 cm/ Bottom Diameter 4.6 cm/ Height 2.6 cm

Preserved in Rui'an Museum

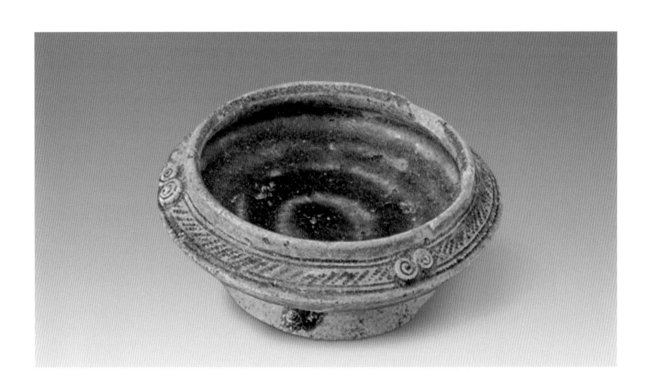

原始青瓷盂

西周晚期

瓷质

口径 8.2 厘米，底径 7 厘米，高 4.4 厘米

瑞安博物馆藏

Primitive Celadon "Yu" (Bowl)

Late Western Zhou Dynasty

Porcelain

Mouth Diameter 8.2 cm/ Bottom Diameter 7 cm/ Height 4.4 cm

Preserved in Rui'an Museum

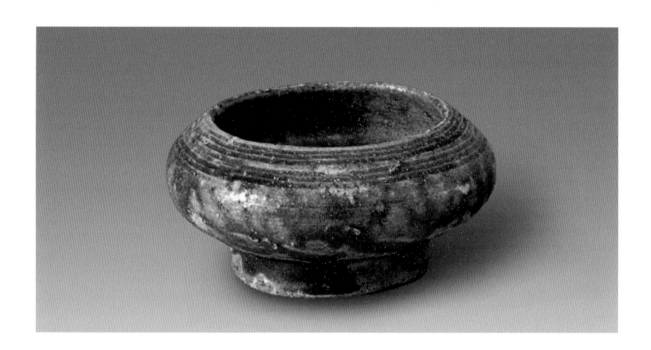

原始青瓷盂

西周晚期

瓷质

口径 6.8 厘米，底径 5.4 厘米，高 4.8 厘米

1992 年浙江省余姚市老虎山一号墩出土。

浙江省文物考古研究所藏

Primitive Celadon "Yu" (Bowl)

Late Western Zhou Dynasty

Porcelain

Mouth Diameter 6.8 cm/ Bottom Diameter 5.4 cm/ Height 4.8 cm

The bowl was unearthed at No.1 Pier in Laohu Mountain, Yuyao City, Zhejiang Province, in the year 1992.

Preserved in Institute of Cultural Relics and Archaeology of Zhejiang Province

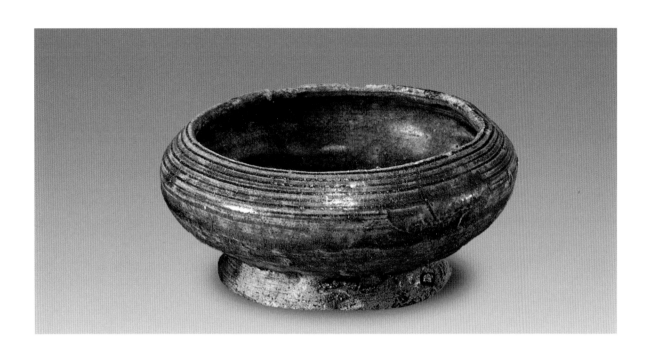

原始青瓷盂

西周晚期

瓷质

口径 7.8 厘米，底径 6.2 厘米，高 4.4 厘米

1992 年浙江省余姚市老虎山一号墩出土。

浙江省文物考古研究所藏

Primitive Celadon "Yu" (Bowl)

Late Western Zhou Dynasty

Porcelain

Mouth Diameter 7.8 cm/ Bottom Diameter 6.2 cm/ Height 4.4 cm

The bowl was unearthed at No.1 Pier in Laohu Mountain, Yuyao City, Zhejiang Province, in the year 1992.

Preserved in Institute of Cultural Relics and Archaeology of Zhejiang Province

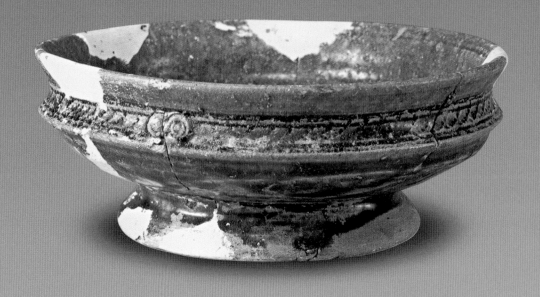

原始青瓷碗

西周晚期春秋初期

瓷质

口径 17.9 厘米，底径 11.4 厘米，高 6.7 厘米

1982 年浙江省长兴便山石室土墩墓出土。

浙江省文物考古研究所藏

Primitive Celadon Bowl

Late Western Zhou Dynasty/ Early Spring and Autumn Period

Porcelain

Mouth Diameter 17.9 cm/ Bottom Diameter 11.4 cm/ Height 6.7 cm

The bowl was unearthed at the mound tomb in Bian Mountain, Shishi Village, Changxing County, Zhejiang Province, in the year 1982.

Preserved in Institute of Cultural Relics and Archaeology of Zhejiang Province

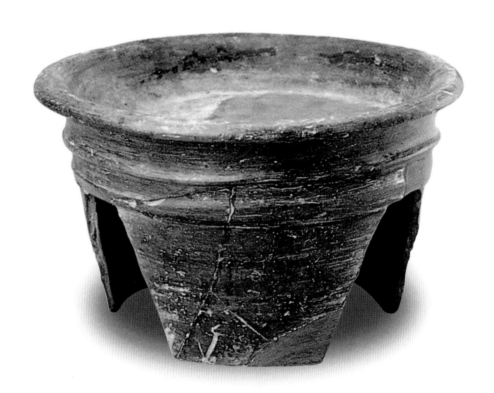

灰陶三足盘

夏文化 (约前 21 世纪—前 16 世纪)

灰陶质

口径 22.5 厘米，高 13.2 厘米

Grey Pottery Tripod Plate

Xia Culture (Circa 21st Century B.C. - 16th Century B.C.)

Grey Pottery

Mouth Diameter 22.5 cm/ Height 13.2 cm

此陶盘在敞口平底的浅盘下附着了三片上宽
下窄的瓦形足，因此又叫瓦足皿，系夏文化
中最有代表意义的器皿之一。功能与陶豆相
同，也是盛食具。河南省洛阳市东干沟遗址
出土。

北京大学赛克勒考古与艺术博物馆藏

Three tile-shaped feet, wide at the top and
narrow at the bottom, are attached to the
openmouthed shallow plate. Therefore, it is
named as the vessel with tile-shaped feet,
which is one of the most typical vessels of the
Xia Culture. Similar to the function of pottery
stemmed bowl, it was used as a food vessel. It
was unearthed from Donggangou Site, Luoyang
City, Henan Province.

Preserved in Arthur M. Sackler Museum of Art
and Archaeology at Peking University

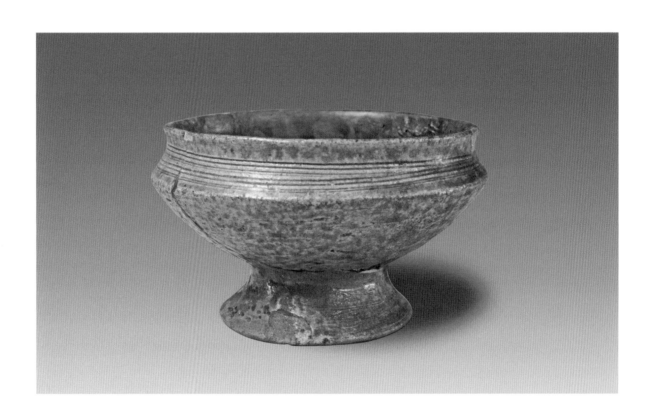

青瓷豆

商

瓷质

口径 12.4 厘米，足径 7.9 厘米，高 7.7 厘米

Celadon "Dou" (Stemmed Bowl)

Shang Dynasty

Porcelain

Mouth Diameter 12.4 cm/ Bottom Diameter 7.9 cm/ Height 7.7 cm

胎质灰白色，烧结程度较好，玻璃质感较强，器内、外施青釉，釉色青中泛灰，胎釉结合紧密，釉面尚明亮。口直微敛，短颈，折肩，腹深内收，圈足较矮。颈部饰不规则的凹弦纹。原始青瓷豆是商周时期典型的食器。1965 年青州市苏埠屯出土。

山东博物馆藏

The greyish white body was fired so intensively that it shows a strong vitreous texture. Both the exterior and interior are covered with bright grayish-green glaze which is closely fitted with the body texture. The bowl has a slightly contracted straight mouth, a short neck, an angular shoulder, a deep belly that is gradually contracted to the bottom, and a relatively short ring foot. Irregular concave strings patterns can be found at the neck. Primitive celadon "Dou" was a typical food container in Shang and Zhou Dynasties. It was unearthed at Sufu Village, Qingzhou City, Shandong Province, in the year 1965.

Preserved in Shandong Museum

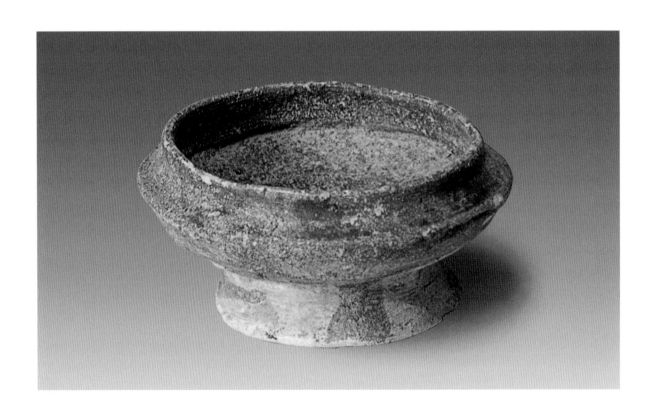

着黑硬陶豆

西周晚期

陶质

口径 7.2 厘米，底径 6.2 厘米，高 4.8 厘米

Black Hard Pottery "Dou" (Stemmed Bowl)

Late Western Zhou Dynasty

Pottery

Mouth Diameter 7.2 cm/ Bottom Diameter 6.2 cm/ Height 4.8 cm

内、外壁均施无光泽的黑色涂层，并可见涂
刷黑层时的流挂现象。

瑞安博物馆藏

Both the exterior and interior of the bowl are
covered with unglazed black coating. Sagging
marks left on the surface during the painting
process remains noticeable.

Preserved in Rui'an Museum

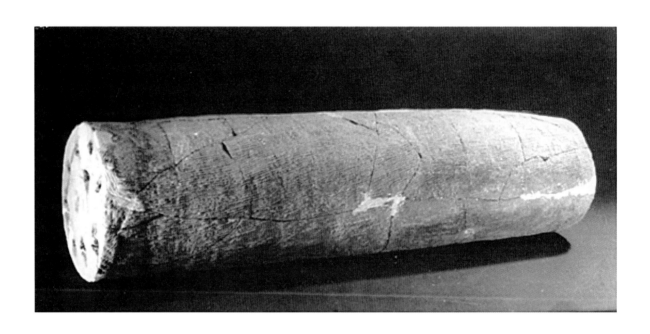

滤孔水道

西周

陶质

长 83 厘米，直径 17.5~21.5 厘米

Water Conduit with Filter Holes

Western Zhou Dynasty

Pottery

Length 83 cm/ Diametre 17.5-21.5 cm

通身绳纹，一端有不规则滤孔十个，用以防止柴草等杂物进入水道。陕西扶风周原遗址出土。

宝鸡市周原博物馆藏

The body is covered with string patterns. At one end are ten irregular filter holes for preventing litters, like firewood and grasses from floating into the water lane. It was unearthed from Zhouyuan Site, Fufeng County, Shaanxi Province. Preserved in Zhouyuan Museum, Baoji City

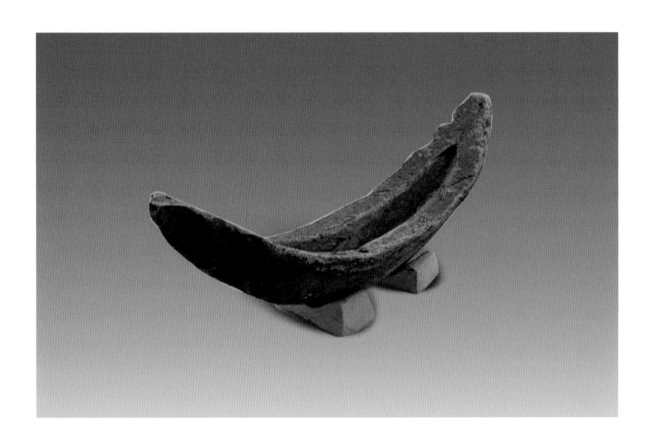

陶药碾

商

陶质

长 36 厘米，宽 10 厘米，高 18 厘米

Pottery Medicine Crusher

Shang Dynasty

Pottery

Length 36 cm/ Width 10 cm/ Height 18 cm

月牙形凹槽，弧形尖底，置于两个凹型底座
上。微残。御生堂传世藏品。此展品说明在
3000 年前的商代已经有形制完备的制药工
具，见证了当时的社会文明进步程度。

北京御生堂中医药博物馆藏

The crescent-shaped groove is welded onto
the concave base and is slightly incomplete.
This artifact is considered as the witness of the
development of Chinese civilization. It is the
evidence of advanced tools of medicine making
in the Shang Dynasty 3,000 years ago. It was
carefully conserved though generations.
Preserved in Chinese Medicine Museum of
Beijing Yu Sheng Tang Drugstore

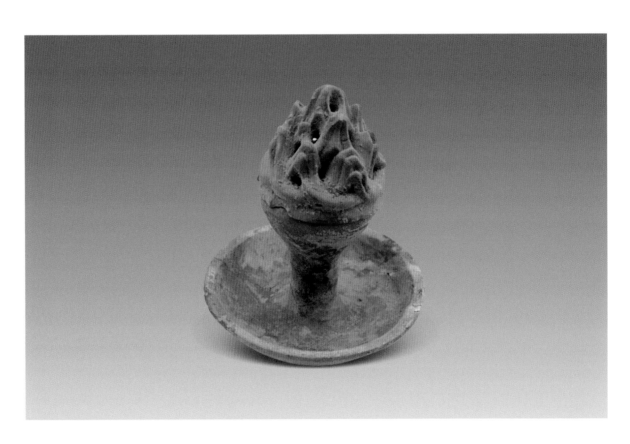

博山香熏

商

陶质

直径 15 厘米，高 18 厘米

Bo Shan Aromatherapy Burner

Shang Dynasty

Pottery

Diameter 15 cm/ Height 18 cm

古人用此物熏烧天然香草料，用于疾病预防和居室卫生，是"治未病"思想和"预防医学"的见证物，是现代香熏疗法的渊源。

北京御生堂中医药博物馆藏

The burner was used for smoking the natural spice, which can prevent disease and enhance indoor sanitation. It is the evidence of the idea of "Disease Prevention" and "Preventive Medicine", and the earliest origin of aromatherapy.

Preserved in Chinese Medicine Museum of Beijing Yu Sheng Tang Drugstore

◇ 第三章　春秋战国

Chapter Three　Spring and Autumn Period and

Warring States Period

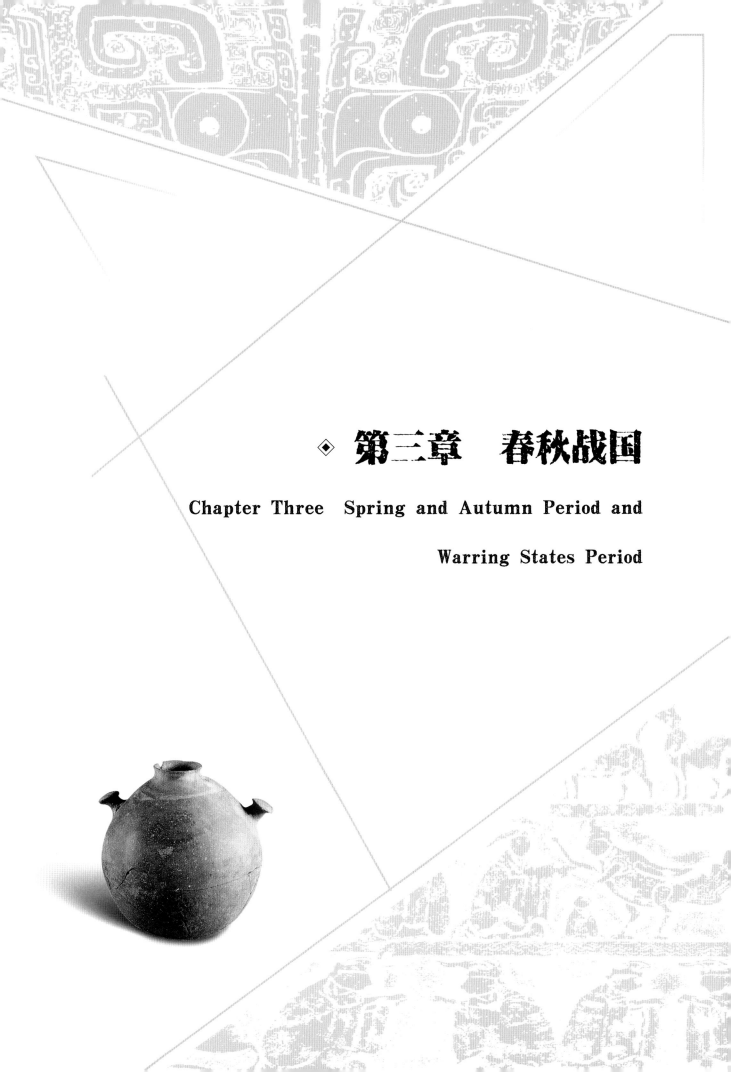

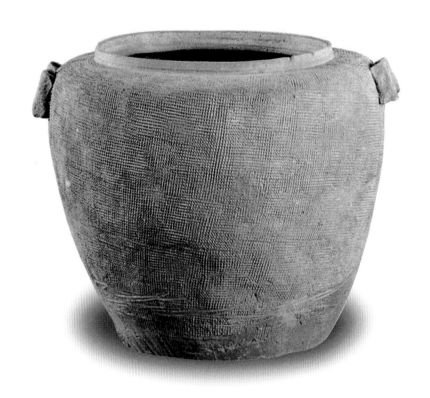

印纹硬陶罐

春秋 (前 770—前 476)

陶质

口径 7.7 厘米，高 9.8 厘米

Stamped Hard Pottery Pot

Spring and Autumn Period (770B.C. ‐476B.C.)

Pottery

Mouth Diameter 7.7 cm/ Height 9.8 cm

河南省固始县侯古堆大墓出土。

河南省文物考古研究院藏

The pot was excavated from Hougudui Tomb in Gushi County, Henan Province.

Preserved in Henan Provincial Institute of Cultural Heritage and Archaeology

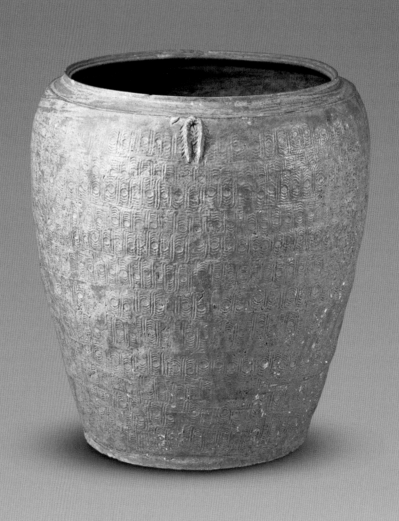

原始瓷罐

春秋

瓷质

口径 23.8 厘米，底径 19.5 厘米，高 30 厘米

口微外撇，束颈，斜折肩，深腹，平底，器肩处贴有一对绚纹耳。施茶黄色青釉，底部露胎。器身拍印圈、线结合的几何纹，由肩至底共十一重。胎质坚硬。

常州博物馆藏

Primitive Porcelain Jar

Spring and Autumn Period

Porcelain

Mouth Diameter 23.8 cm/ Bottom Diameter 19.5 cm/ Height 30 cm

The jar, coated with celadon glaze in tawny yellow colour, has a slightly flared mouth, a contracted neck, a tilting angular shoulder, a deep belly and a flat bottom where the hard body is exposed. The body of the utensil is stamped from the shoulder to the bottom with eleven tiers of geometric designs that combine circles and lines. A pair of ears with string designs is attached to the shoulder.

Preserved in Changzhou Museum

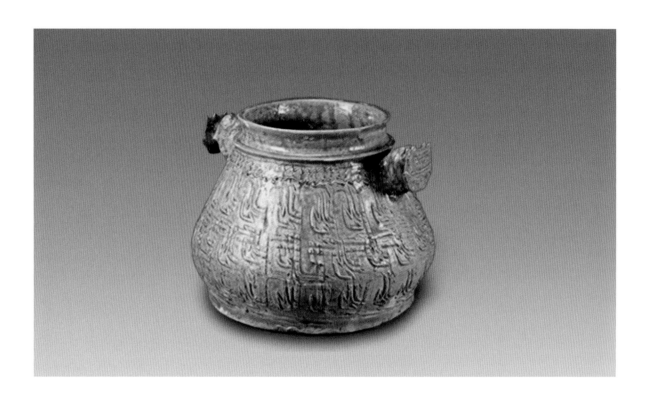

原始瓷罐

春秋

瓷质

口径 13.5 厘米，底径 19 厘米，高 17.1 厘米

Primitive Porcelain Jar

Spring and Autumn Period

Porcelain

Mouth Diameter 13.5 cm/ Bottom Diameter 19 cm/ Height 17.1 cm

口沿外折，短颈，溜肩，鼓腹，平底，肩部
有两个鋬耳。内、外施茶黄色釉，底部无釉，
胎体较坚致，颈部饰一圈凸棱和数周锯齿形
刻划纹，腹部拍印双线勾联纹。

常州博物馆藏

The jar, coated with celadon glaze in tawny
yellow colour both on the exterior and the
interior, has a upturned mouth rim, a short neck,
a tilting shoulder, a bulging body and a flat
bottom where the hard body is exposed. On the
shoulder is a pair of handles. Around the neck is
found a raised ridge together with several tiers
of saw-toothed designs. Around the stomach
are stamped double-lined linked hook patterns.
Preserved in Changzhou Museum

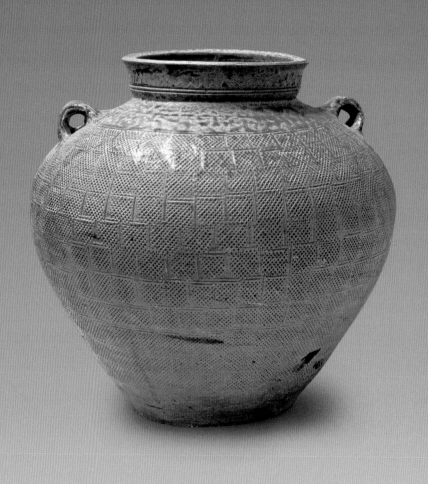

青釉双系罐

战国

瓷质

口径 14.8 厘米，底径 13.7 厘米，高 28.2 厘米

直口微侈，矮颈，颈上一周刻画水波纹与弦纹，溜肩，鼓腹向下渐收，腹部上有对称竖耳一对。施釉不到底。罐身拍印几何形印纹。造型规整，纹饰清晰，全器集实用、美观于一身。江苏省江宁区湖熟镇出土。

南京市博物馆藏

Celadon Jar with Double Loop Handles

Warring States Period

Porcelain

Mouth Diameter 14.8 cm/ Bottom Diameter 13.7 cm/ Height 28.2 cm

The jar has a straight and slightly flared mouth, a short neck with incised water ripples and bowstring designs, a sloping shoulder, a swelling stomach gradually tapering downwards, to which is attached a pair of symmetrical prick ears, and an unglazed bottom. The body of the jar is decorated with geometrical designs. With neat structure and clear designs, the jar is of both functional and aesthetic values. It was excavated from Hushu Town, Jiangning District, Jiangsu Province.

Preserved in Nanjing Municipal Museum

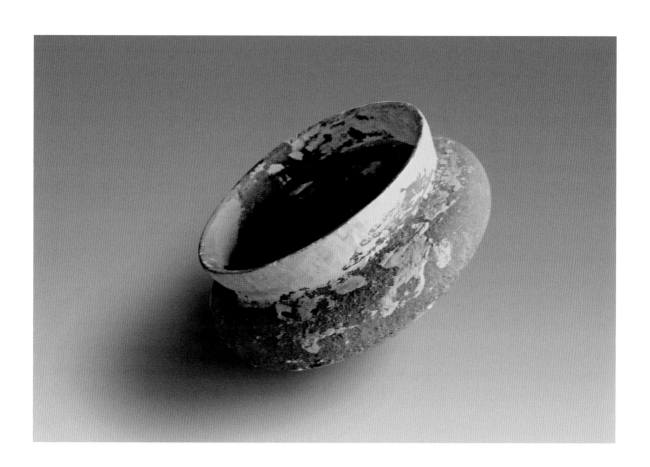

尖底罐

战国

陶质

口径 7.5 厘米，高 5.5 厘米

Jar with Pointed Bottom

Warring States Period

Pottery

Mouth Diameter 7.5 cm/ Height 5.5 cm

稍残。由成都市考古队调拨。

成都中医药大学中医药传统文化博物馆藏

The jar was slightly damaged and was allocated from the archaeological team of Chengdu.

Preserved in Museum of Traditional Chinese Medicine Culture, Chengdu University of Traditional Chinese Medicine

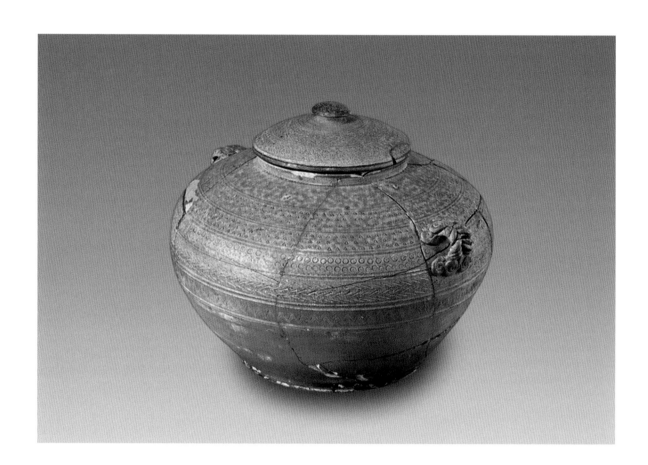

原始青瓷圈足瓿

战国晚期

瓷质

口径 14.4 厘米，底径 18.4 厘米，高 29.8 厘米

Primitive Celadon "Bu" (Jar) with Ring Foot

Late Warring States Period

Porcelain

Mouth Diameter 14.4 cm/ Bottom Diameter 18.4 cm/ Height 29.8 cm

1992 年浙江省余姚老虎山一号墩出土。

浙江省文物考古研究所藏

The jar was excavated from No.1 Pier in Laohu
Mountain, Yuyao City, Zhejiang Province, in
the year 1992.
Preserved in Institute of Cultural Relics and
Archaeology of Zhejiang Province

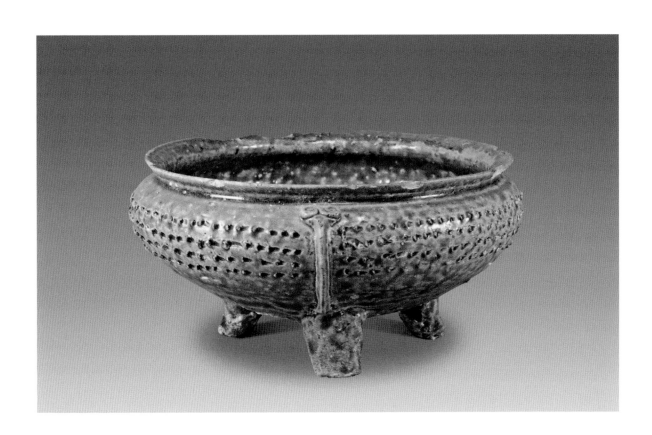

原始瓷鼎

春秋

瓷质

口径 17.9 厘米，腹径 18.8 厘米，高 9.5 厘米

Primitive Pottery "Ding" (Tripod)

Spring and Autumn Period

Porcelain

Mouth Diameter 17.9 cm/ Belly Diametre 18.8 cm/ Height 9.5 cm

侈口，束颈，浅圆腹，三足粗短。胎体坚致，釉色茶黄。腹部装饰四排锥刺纹，并堆塑三条竖向扉棱与三足相连，扉棱顶端各饰一 S 形堆纹。器内壁见不规则螺旋纹。

常州博物馆藏

The "Ding", covered with tawny yellow glaze, has a hard body, a wide flared mouth, a contracted neck, a flat swelling stomach and three stubby feet. The belly is decorated with four tiers of pricks patterns, with three vertical ridges in relief moulded on it as well. The ridges reach the three feet. The top of each ridge is adorned with an S-shaped pattern. On the interior wall can be seen irregular spiral patterns.

Preserved in Changzhou Museum

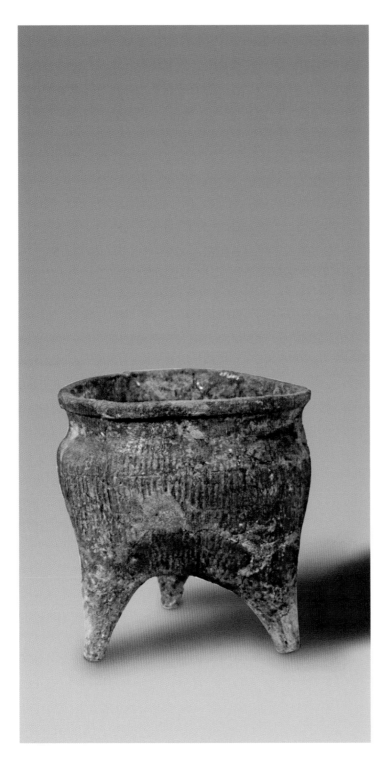

陶鬲

春秋

陶质

口径 17 厘米，通高 17 厘米，裆高
5 厘米

Pottery "Li" (Cauldron)

Spring and Autumn Period

Pottery

Mouth Diameter 17 cm/ Height 17 cm/

Crotch Height 5 cm

饮食容器。江苏六合区程桥镇程桥中学校址
出土。

南京博物院藏

The tripod served as a food vessel. It was
excavated from Chengqiao Middle School of
Chengqiao Town in Liuhe District, Jiangsu
Province.
Preserved in Nanjing Museum

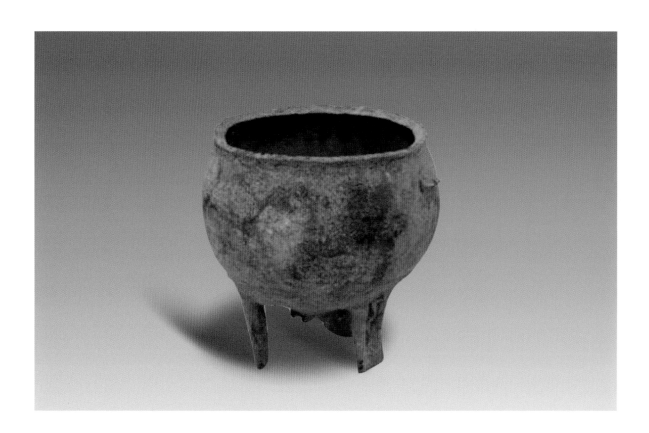

陶鬲

战国

黑陶质

口径 22 厘米，通高 30 厘米，足高 8 厘米

Pottery Tripod

Warring States Period

Black Pottery

Mouth Diameter 22 cm/ Height 30 cm/ Foot Height 8 cm

侈口，束颈，鼓腹，三足。煮药器皿。

北京御生堂中医药博物馆藏

The tripod has a widely flared mouth, a contracted neck, a bulged belly and three feet. It was a tool of boiling medicine.

Preserved in Chinese Medicine Museum of Beijing Yu Sheng Tang Drugstore

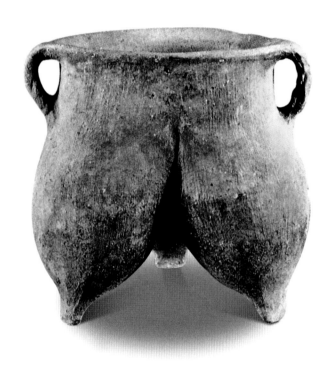

夹砂灰陶双耳鬲

战国（约前 475—前 221）

夹砂灰陶质

腹径 20.5 厘米，高 19.5 厘米

Grey Sandy Pottery Tripod "Li" (Cauldron) with Double Handles

Warring States Period (Circa 475 B.C.—221 B.C.)

Grey Sandy Pottery

Belly Diametre 20.5 cm/ Height 19.5 cm

这种形态的陶鬲在中原地区的古代文化中极少见到，它与中原陶鬲有着不同的文化渊源，是春秋战国之际西部戎人的典型器具。陕西省宝鸡市出土。

北京大学赛克勒考古与艺术博物馆藏

Tripod "Li" in this shape has rarely been seen in the ancient culture of Central China. Originating from a culture distinct from that of the tripod in Central China, this tripod was a typical utensil used by tribes in the west border areas during the Periods of Spring-autumn and Warring States. It was excavated in Baoji City, Shaanxi Province.

Preserved in Arthur M. Sackler Museum of Art and Archaeology at Peking University

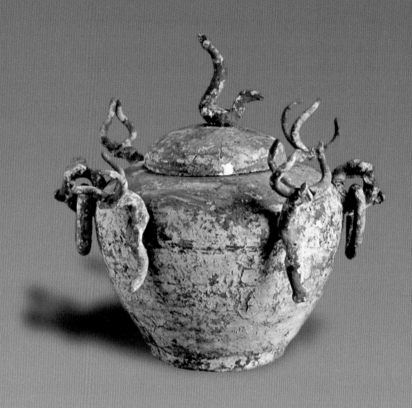

陶罍

战国

陶质

口径 9.9 厘米，腹径 23 厘米，通高 28.6 厘米

湖北省文物考古研究所藏

Pottery Urn-shaped "Lei" (Wine Vessel)

Warring States Period

Pottery

Mouth Diameter 9.9 cm/ Belly Diametre 23 cm/ Height 28.6 cm

Preserved in Hubei Provincial Institute of Cultural Relics and Archaeology

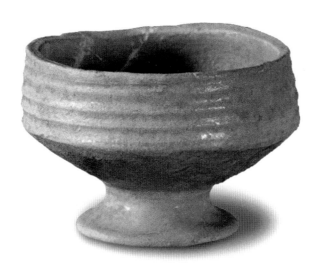

青釉陶豆

战国

陶质

口径 10.2 厘米，底径 6.3 厘米，腹深 5 厘米，高 7.2 厘米

江苏无锡市荣巷 M28 号墓出土。

南京博物院藏

Celadon Pottery "Dou" (Stemmed Cup)

Warring States Period

Pottery

Mouth Diameter 10.2 cm/ Bottom Diameter 6.3 cm/ Depth 5 cm/ Height 7.2 cm

The cup was excavated from M28 Tomb of Rongxiang Village in Wuxi City, Jiangsu Province.

Preserved in Nanjing Museum

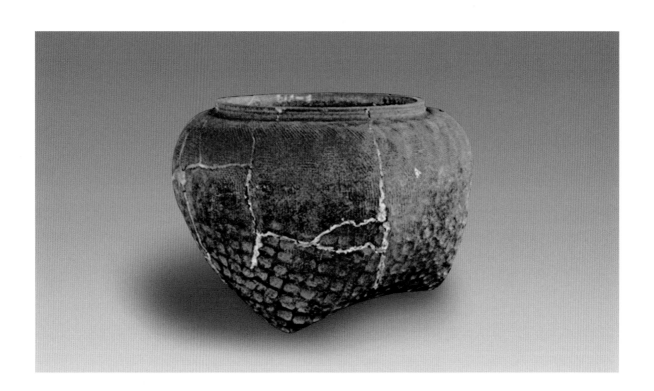

大陶釜

战国

陶质

口径 31 厘米，底径 36 厘米，通高 33 厘米，重 1700 克

Big Pottery "Fu" (Cauldron)

Warring States Period

Pottery

Mouth Diameter 31 cm/ Bottom Diameter 36 cm/ Height 33 cm/ Weight 1,700 g

直口，直腹，三袋状足。上腹为绳纹，下腹
为方块纹。炊器。有修补。

陕西医史博物馆藏

The cauldron has a straight mouth, a straight
body and three pouch-shaped feet. On the
upper belly are carved string patterns, while on
the lower belly a square pattern. The cooking
utensil has been repaired.

Preserved in Shaanxi Museum of Medical History

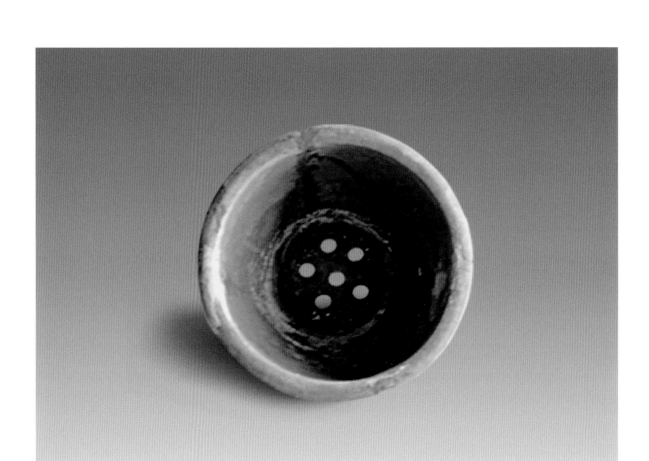

甑

战国

陶质

口径 7 厘米，高 23 厘米

"Zeng" (Steamer)

Warring States Period

Pottery

Mouth Diameter 7 cm/ Height 23 cm

底部有五个圆孔，为蒸煮用具。由成都市考
古队调拨。

　　成都中医药大学中医药传统文化博物馆藏

The caldron has five circular holes on the
bottom and was used for steaming food. It
was allocated from the archaeological team of
Chengdu.
Preserved in Museum of Traditional Chinese
Medicine Culture, Chengdu University of
Traditional Chinese Medicine

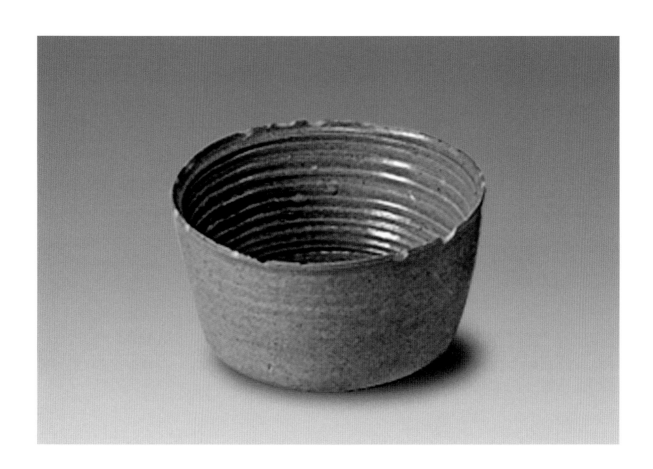

原始青瓷碗

春秋中晚期

瓷质

口径 8.8 厘米，底径 4.8 厘米，高 5 厘米

Primitive Celadon Bowl

Mid-late Spring and Autumn Period

Porcelain

Mouth Diameter 8.8 cm/ Bottom Diameter 4.8 cm/ Height 5 cm

1982 年浙江省长兴县便山土墩墓出土。

浙江省文物考古研究所藏

The bowl was excavated from the mound
tomb in Bian Mountain in Changxing County,
Zhejiang Province, in the year 1982.
Preserved in Institute of Cultural Relics and
Archaeology of Zhejiang Province

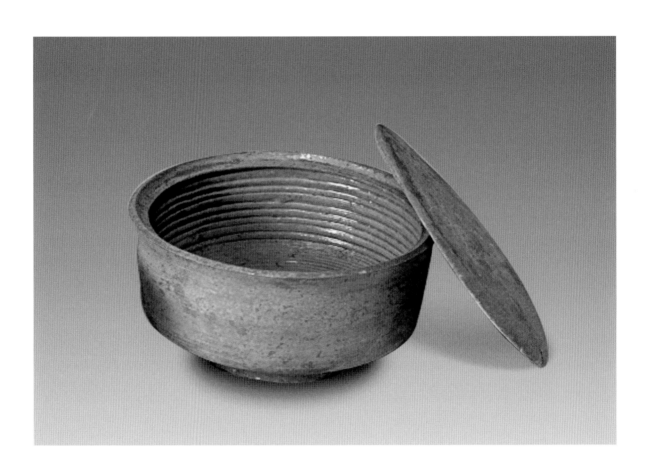

原始青瓷碗

春秋中晚期

瓷质

直径 11.4 厘米，底径 6.2 厘米，高 6.3 厘米

Primitive Celadon Bowl

Mid-late Spring and Autumn Period

Porcelain

Diameter 11.4 cm/ Bottom Diameter 6.2 cm/ Height 6.3 cm

1982 年浙江省长兴县便山土墩墓出土。

浙江省文物考古研究所藏

The bowl was excavated from the mound
tomb in Bian Mountain in Changxing County,
Zhejiang Province, in the year 1982.
Preserved in Institute of Cultural Relics and
Archaeology of Zhejiang Province

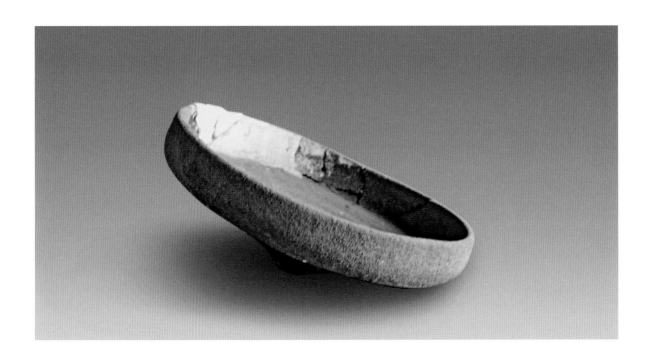

尖底盘

战国

陶质

口径 12 厘米，高 4 厘米

稍残。由成都市考古队调拨。

成都中医药大学中医药传统文化博物馆藏

Plate with Pointed Bottom

Warring States Period

Pottery

Mouth Diameter 12 cm/ Height 4 cm

The plate is slightly damaged. It was allocated from the archaeological team of Chengdu.

Preserved in Museum of Traditional Chinese Medicine Culture, Chengdu University of Traditional Chinese Medicine

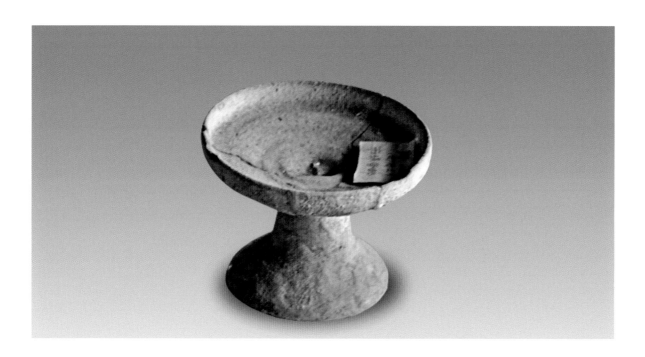

盒

战国

陶质

口径 10 厘米，高 7 厘米

高圈足。由成都市考古队调拨。

成都中医药大学中医药传统文化博物馆藏

Box

Warring States Period

Pottery

Mouth Diameter 10 cm/ Height 7 cm

The box has a stem ring foot. It was allocated from the archaeological team of Chengdu.

Preserved in Museum of Traditional Chinese Medicine Culture, Chengdu University of Traditional Chinese Medicine

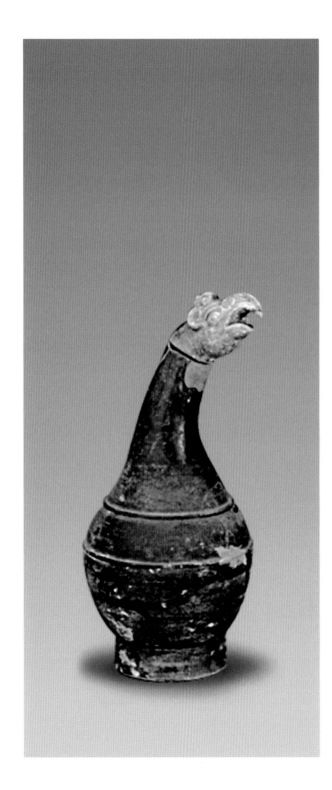

鸟盖匏形陶壶

战国

陶质

口径 4 厘米，高 30 厘米

Gourd-shaped Bottle with a Bird Lid

Warring States Period

Pottery

Mouth Diameter 4 cm/ Height 30 cm

壶体似匏形，长斜颈，椭圆形腹，盖为鸟首状，鸟尖嘴圆目，形象凶猛。匏壶，古代酒器之一，西周、战国墓葬有青铜匏形壶出土，其形制与此壶大体相似。此壶姿态窈窕，制作精致。

山西博物院藏

The bottle is in the shape of a gourd, with a long sloping neck and an oval belly. The lid resembles a fierce looking bird's head with sharp mouth and round eyes. The gourd-shaped bottle is a typical ancient wine vessel. Some bronze gourd-shaped bottles unearthed from tombs of Western Zhou and Warring States Period are similar to this one in shape. This bottle displays an elegant shape and exquisite craftsmanship.

Preserved in Shanxi Museum

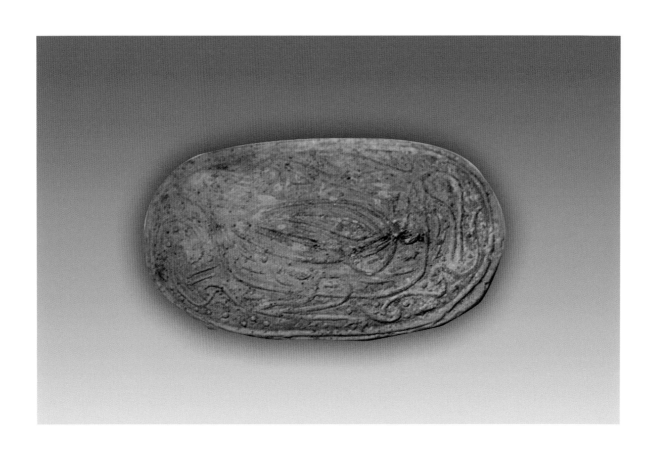

陶砭

战国

陶质

长 15 厘米，宽 8 厘米，高 2 厘米

Pottery Bian

Warring States Period

Pottery

Length 15 cm/ Width 8 cm/ Height 2 cm

椭圆形，正、反面均有精美的图案。砭中空，手摇可"哗哗"作响，加热后其热度可长时间不散，用于挤压伤口、缓解病痛以及作为按摩、刮痧的医疗保健用具。砭石疗法是最早的治疗疾病的方法，《史记·扁鹊仓公列传》中生动地记载了扁鹊用砭救治虢国太子和秦武王面部痈肿的故事。

北京御生堂中医药博物馆藏

The elliptical bian with empty inner part has the exquisite motifs on both sides. It can make "Bibi" sound when shook and the heat can be kept for a long time. It was used for squeezing the wound, relieving the pain，and medical and health care appliance for massage and scraping. The therapy of stone bian is the earliest treatment in the history of traditional Chinese medicine. The biography of Bian Que in *Historical Records* vividly recorded how Bian Que cured the prince of Guo Country and the Emperor Wu of Qin Dynasty by bian treatment. Preserved in Chinese Medicine Museum of Beijing Yu Sheng Tang Drugstore

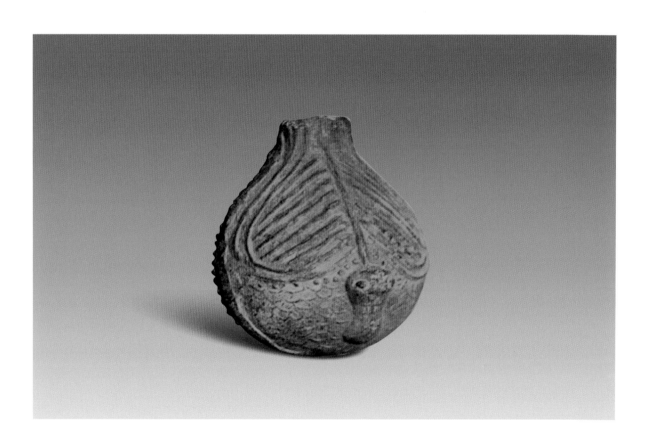

陶砭

战国

陶质

长 12 厘米，宽 9 厘米，高 2 厘米

Pottery Bian

Warring States Period

Pottery

Length 12 cm/ Width 9 cm/ Height 2 cm

鸟形，图案精美。砭中空，手摇可"哗哗"作响，加热后其热度可长时间不散，用于挤压伤口、缓解病痛以及作为按摩、刮痧的医疗保健用具。砭石疗法是最早的治疗疾病的方法，《史记·扁鹊仓公列传》中生动地记载了扁鹊用砭救治虢国太子和秦武王面部痈肿的故事。

北京御生堂中医药博物馆藏

The Bian with empty inner part is shaped like a bird and is carved with the exquisite patterns. It can make "Bibi" sound when shook and the heat can be kept for a long time. It was used for squeezing the wound, relieving the pain，and medical and health care appliance for massage and scraping. The therapy of stone bian is the earliest treatment in the history of traditional Chinese medicine. The biography of Bian Que in *Historical Records* vividly recorded how Bian Que cured the prince of Guo Country and the Emperor Wu of Qin Dynasty by bian treatment.

Preserved in Chinese Medicine Museum of Beijing Yu Sheng Tang Drugstore

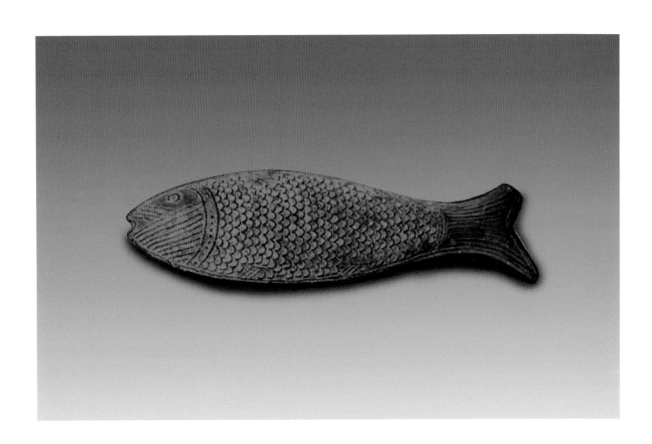

陶砭

战国

陶质

长 20 厘米，宽 5 厘米，高 2 厘米

Pottery Bian

Warring States Period

Pottery

Length 20 cm/ Width 5 cm/ Height 2 cm

鱼形，图案精美。砭中空，手摇可"哗哗"作响，加热后其热度可长时间不散，用于挤压伤口、缓解病痛以及作为按摩、刮痧的医疗保健用具。砭石疗法是最早的治疗疾病的方法，《史记·扁鹊仓公列传》中生动地记载了扁鹊用砭救治虢国太子和秦武王面部痈肿的故事。

北京御生堂中医药博物馆藏

The bian with empty inner part is shaped like a fish and is carved with the exquisite patterns. It can make "Bibi" sound when shook and the heat can be kept for a long time. It was used for squeezing the wound, relieving the pain，and medical and health care appliance for massage and scraping. The therapy of stone bian is the earliest treatment in the history of traditional Chinese medicine. The biography of Bian Que in *Historical Records* vividly recorded how Bian Que cured the prince of Guo Country and the Emperor Wu of Qin Dynasty by bian treatment.

Preserved in Chinese Medicine Museum of Beijing Yu Sheng Tang Drugstore

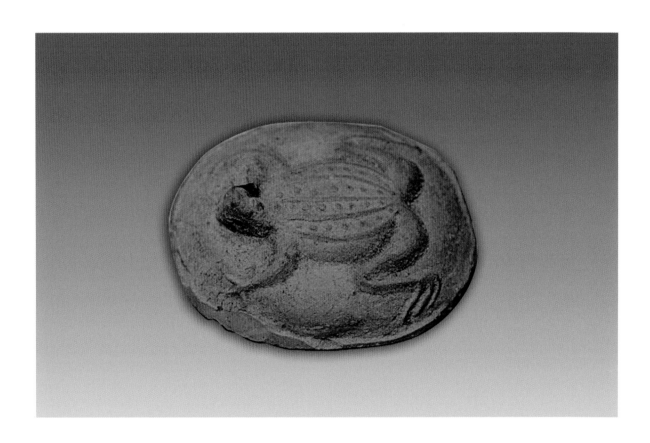

陶砭

战国

陶质

长 10 厘米，宽 9 厘米，高 2 厘米

Pottery Bian

Warring States Period

Pottery

Length 10 cm/ Width 9 cm/ Height 2 cm

椭圆形，上塑蛙形图案。砭中空，手摇可"哗哗"作响，加热后其热度可长时间不散，用于挤压伤口、缓解病痛以及作为按摩、刮痧的医疗保健用具。砭石疗法是最早的治疗疾病的方法，《史记·扁鹊仓公列传》中生动地记载了扁鹊用砭救治虢国太子和秦武王面部痈肿的故事。

北京御生堂中医药博物馆藏

The elliptical bian with hollow belly is decorated with a frog. It can make "Bibi" sound when shook and the heat can be kept for a long time. It was used for squeezing the wound, relieving the pain, and medical and health care appliance for massage and scraping. The therapy of stone bian is the earliest treatment in the history of traditional Chinese medicine. The biography of Bian Que in *Historical Records* vividly recorded how Bian Que cured the prince of Guo Country and the Emperor Wu of Qin Dynasty by bian treatment.

Preserved in Chinese Medicine Museum of Beijing Yu Sheng Tang Drugstore

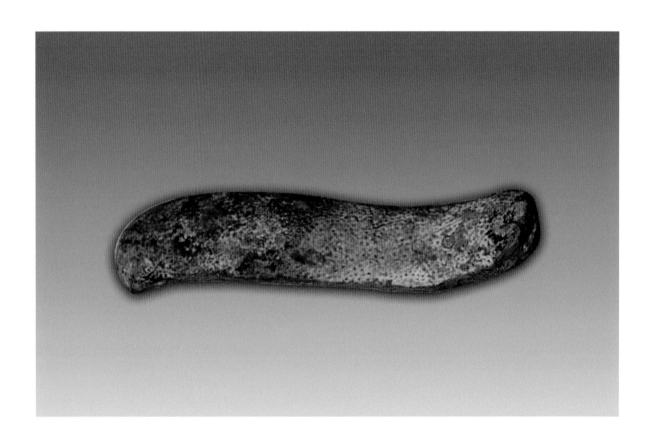

陶砭

战国

陶质

长 22 厘米，宽 4 厘米，高 2 厘米

Pottery Bian

Warring States Period

Pottery

Length 22 cm/ Width 4 cm/ Height 2 cm

S 形，正、反面均有精美的图案。砭中空，手摇可"哗哗"作响，加热后其热度可长时间不散，用于挤压伤口、缓解病痛以及作为按摩、刮痧的医疗保健用具。砭石疗法是最早的治疗疾病的方法，《史记·扁鹊仓公列传》中生动地记载了扁鹊用砭救治虢国太子和秦武王面部痈肿的故事。

北京御生堂中医药博物馆藏

The S-shaped bian with empty inner part is decorated with a frog. It can make "Bibi" sound when shook and the heat can be kept for a long time. It was used for squeezing the wound, relieving the pain, and medical and health care appliance for massage and scraping. The therapy of stone bian is the earliest treatment in the history of traditional Chinese medicine. The biography of Bian Que in *Historical Records* vividly recorded how Bian Que cured the prince of Guo Country and the Emperor Wu of Qin Dynasty by bian treatment.

Preserved in Chinese Medicine Museum of Beijing Yu Sheng Tang Drugstore

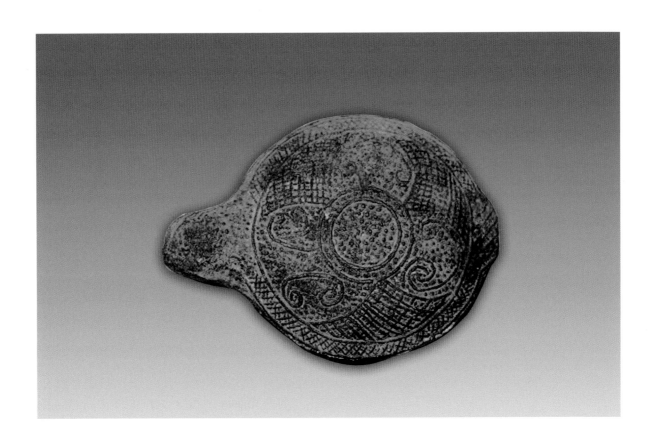

陶砭

战国

陶质

长8厘米，宽6厘米，高3厘米

Pottery Bian

Warring States Period

Pottery

Length 8 cm/ Width 6 cm/ Height 3cm

龟形，正、反面均有精美的图案。砭中空，手摇可"哗哗"作响，加热后其热度可长时间不散，用于挤压伤口、缓解病痛以及作为按摩、刮痧的医疗保健用具。砭石疗法是最早的治疗疾病的方法，《史记·扁鹊仓公列传》中生动地记载了扁鹊用砭救治虢国太子和秦武王面部痈肿的故事。

北京御生堂中医药博物馆藏

The bian with hollow belly is shaped like a turtle and is carved with the exquisite patterns on both sides. It can make "Bibi" sound when shook and the heat can be kept for a long time. It was used for squeezing the wound, relieving the pain，and medical and health care appliance for massage and scraping. The therapy of stone bian is the earliest treatment in the history of traditional Chinese medicine. The biography of Bian Que in *Historical Records* vividly recorded how Bian Que cured the prince of Guo Country and Emperor Wu of Qin Dynasty by using the bian.

Preserved in Chinese Medicine Museum of Beijing Yu Sheng Tang Drugstore

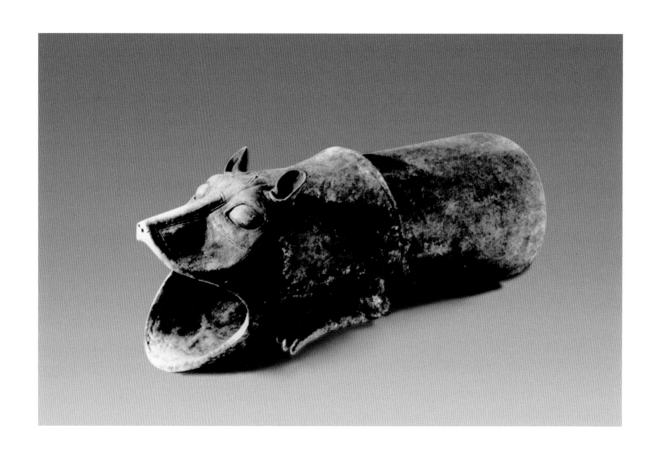

虎头形陶水管口

战国

陶质

Tigerhead-shaped Water Pipe Outlet

Warring States Period

Pottery

管道前端呈虎头状，竖耳瞠目，口部大张，两腿平伸。其后接圆管小于虎头管口，形成子口，便于套接。此器为排水管道的排水口。1958 年于河北省易县燕下都遗址出土。

中国国家博物馆藏

The front end of the pipe is in the shape of a tiger head with prick ears, beady eyes, a wide open mouth and horizontally extended legs. The round pipe attached to the front one is made smaller in size in order to form a socket. This ware is a drain outlet which was excavated from the ruins of Secondary Capital of Yan in Yi County, Hebei Province, in the year 1958.

Preserved in National Museum of China

索 引

（馆藏地按拼音字母排序）

Index

参考文献

[1] 李经纬 . 中国古代医史图录 [M]. 北京：人民卫生出版社，1992.

[2] 傅维康，李经纬，林昭庚 . 中国医学通史：文物图谱卷 [M]. 北京：人民卫生出版社，2000.

[3] 和中浚，吴鸿洲 . 中华医学文物图集 [M]. 成都：四川人民出版社，2001.

[4] 上海中医药博物馆 . 上海中医药博物馆馆藏珍品 [M]. 上海：上海科学技术出版社，2013.

[5] 西藏自治区博物馆 . 西藏博物馆 [M]. 北京：五洲传播出版社，2005.

[6] 崔乐泉 . 中国古代体育文物图录：中英文本 [M]. 北京：中华书局，2000.

[7] 张金明，陆雪春 . 中国古铜镜鉴赏图录 [M]. 北京：中国民族摄影艺术出版社，2002.

[8] 文物精华编辑委员会 . 文物精华 [M]. 北京：文物出版社，1964.

[9] 谭维四 . 湖北出土文物精华 [M]. 武汉：湖北教育出版社，2001.

[10] 常州市博物馆 . 常州文物精华 [M]. 北京：文物出版社，1998.

[11] 镇江博物馆 . 镇江文物精华 [M]. 合肥：黄山书社，1997.

[12] 贵州省文化厅，贵州省博物馆 . 贵州文物精华 [M]. 贵阳：贵州人民出版社，2005.

[13] 徐良玉 . 扬州馆藏文物精华 [M]. 南京：江苏古籍出版社，2001.

[14] 昭陵博物馆，陕西历史博物馆 . 昭陵文物精华 [M]. 西安：陕西人民美术出版社，1991.

[15] 南通博物苑 . 南通博物苑文物精华 [M]. 北京：文物出版社，2005.

[16] 邯郸市文物研究所 . 邯郸文物精华 [M]. 北京：文物出版社，2005.

[17] 张秀生，刘友恒，聂连顺，等 . 中国河北正定文物精华 [M]. 北京：文化艺术出版社，1998.

[18] 陕西省咸阳市文物局 . 咸阳文物精华 [M]. 北京：文物出版社，2002.

[19] 安阳市文物管理局 . 安阳文物精华 [M]. 北京：文物出版社，2004.

[20] 深圳市博物馆 . 深圳市博物馆文物精华 [M]. 北京：文物出版社，1998.

[21]《中国文物精华》编辑委员会 . 中国文物精华（1993）[M]. 北京：文物出版社，1993.

[22] 夏路，刘永生.山西省博物馆馆藏文物精华 [M].太原：山西人民出版社，1999.

[23] 文物精华编辑委员会.文物精华 [M].北京：文物出版社，1957.

[24] 山西博物院，湖北省博物馆.荆楚长歌：九连墩楚墓出土文物精华 [M].太原：山西人民出版社，2011.

[25] 刘广堂，石金鸣，宋建忠.晋国雄风：山西出土两周文物精华 [M].沈阳：万卷出版公司，2009.

[26] 沈君山，王国平，单迎红.滦平博物馆馆藏文物精华 [M].北京：中国文联出版社，2012.

[27] 张家口市博物馆.张家口市博物馆馆藏文物精华 [M].北京：科学出版社，2011.

[28] 浙江省文物考古研究所.浙江考古精华 [M].北京：文物出版社，1999.

[29] 故宫博物院.故宫雕刻珍萃 [M].北京：紫禁城出版社，2004.

[30] 故宫博物院紫禁城出版社.故宫博物院藏宝录 [M].上海：上海文艺出版社，1986.

[31] 首都博物馆.大元三都 [M].北京：科学出版社，2016.

[32] 新疆维吾尔自治区博物馆.新疆出土文物 [M].北京：文物出版社，1975.

[33] 王兴伊，段逸山.新疆出土涉医文书辑校 [M].上海：上海科学技术出版社，2016.

[34] 刘学春.刍议医药卫生文物的概念与分类标准 [J].中华中医药杂志，2016，31（11）:4406-4409.

[35] 上海古籍出版社.中国艺海 [M].上海：上海古籍出版社，1994.

[36] 紫都，岳鑫.一生必知的 200 件国宝 [M].呼和浩特：远方出版社，2005.

[37] 谭维四.湖北出土文物精华 [M].武汉：湖北教育出版社，2001.

[38] 张建青.青海彩陶收藏与鉴赏 [M].北京：中国文史出版社，2007.

[39] 银景琦.仡佬族文物 [M].南宁：广西人民出版社，2014.

[40] 廖果，梁峻，李经纬.东西方医学的反思与前瞻 [M].北京：中医古籍出版社，2002.

[41] 梁峻，张志斌，廖果，等.中华医药文明史集论 [M].北京：中医古籍出版社，2003.

[42] 郑蓉，庄乾竹，刘聪，等.中国医药文化遗产考论 [M].北京：中医古籍出版社，2005.